what people are saying about
worth the ride

A refreshingly humorous and forthright account of life with a supposedly debilitating disease. Josh invites you into his life and shows you around with such candor that before you know it, he's a sarcastic, ambitious, sensitive old friend whose crushes on girls and competitiveness in the classroom are far more salient characteristics of his personhood than the wheelchair or the physical limitations. Thank you, Josh, for telling it like it is!

—*Tracy Kramer Seckler,*
Co-founder of Charley's Fund

A vivid description of the courage and fortitude of a young man's journey with Duchenne muscular dystrophy. It is a song of triumph and a testimony on how one can take control of the uncontrollable.

—*Richard S. Finkel, M.D.,*
Director, Neuromuscular Program at
The Children's Hospital of Philadelphia

I met Josh when he was 12 years old, at which time I was fortunate to become part of this special young boy's journey. Now 29, Josh writes that it's unlikely he will be alive when a cure for Duchenne muscular dystrophy is found. This is so untrue ... Josh continues to touch others fighting this battle, finding and sharing an emotional bond, physical strength and the courage to stand up to this devastating disease. Josh is a true champion, and to all those Philly fans in search of a championship ... you found your winner ... Josh Winheld, who will forever live in your hearts.

—*John Bolaris,*
Chief Meteorologist, Fox 29 News

The book, like his Winheld's World blog, opens a window into the mind of a sensitive, hard-charging soul who happens to have used a wheelchair since age 10, and who knows that time is precious.

—*Excerpt from* "Aspirations Like Any Other,"
Daniel Rubin, The Philadelphia Inquirer

worth the ride

worth the ride

the ride

My Journey with Duchenne Muscular Dystrophy

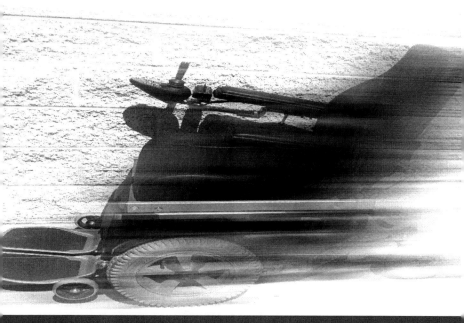

Josh Winheld

an autobiography

Worth the Ride:
My Journey with Duchenne Muscular Dystrophy;
An Autobiography
Josh Winheld

Worth the Ride: My Journey with Duchenne Muscular Dystrophy;
An Autobiography Copyright © 2008 by Josh Winheld.

Cover and interior design by Pneuma Books, LLC
www.pneumabooks.com

ISBN 13: 978-0-9814571-0-9
LCCN: 2008921951

PRINTED IN THE UNITED STATES OF AMERICA
on acid-free paper ∞

16 15 14 13 12 10 09 08   01 02 03 04 05 06 07 08

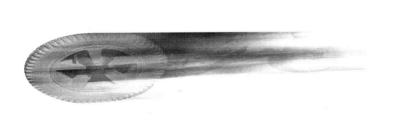

Contents

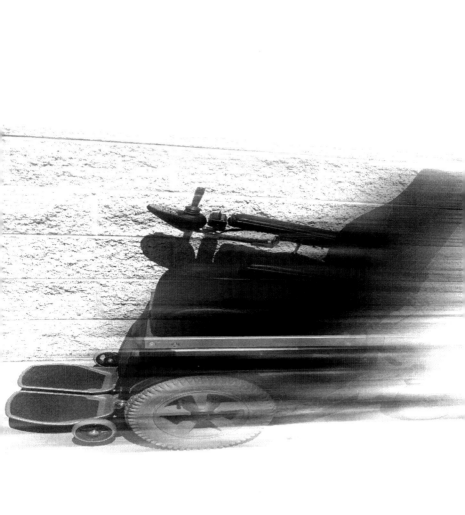

Foreword

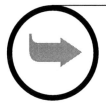

When the door closes, find a window. Duchenne closes doors. There is no treatment. No cure.

Duchenne is lethal. Boys with Duchenne are typically diagnosed between two and five years of age. It is predicted they will die before reaching 30. I have heard it said that you cannot die well over 20+ years. It's true. But you can live well for 20+ years. It is a choice.

When your son is diagnosed with Duchenne muscular dystrophy, it is hard to know what to do, what to say to him, what to say to anyone. You saw something early on. He did not keep up with his little friends. His calf muscles were big, bigger than other boys. Your friends noticed. They may have made offhanded comments about his big calf muscles, "football player muscles."

The diagnosis arrives with a description. Duchenne, a sex-linked disorder that primarily affects boys. This disease is caused by a mutation in a gene that produces an important muscle protein. Without this fully functional protein, muscle cells cannot survive. This is often not detected until parents notice something is different, difficulty walking or running, trouble walking up steps or speech delay. Duchenne is characterized by a progressive loss of strength. Teenage boys with this disease are unable to walk, and if they reach their late teens the ability to move their arms is lost. Duchenne is fatal, 100 percent.

There are no words for a parent to explain, to understand. The diagnosis is difficult to grasp for parents and family members. How could this happen? Why? What will life be like for him? Will he be happy? Parents think about what to say, what words to use. They wonder what their son is thinking, how much he knows, and if he understands the words, "100 percent fatal."

Questions are hard to ask because we want to protect our sons. Dying is not an easy subject. At the same time we want to know what they think, how they feel. Maybe we are afraid to know.

My sons were diagnosed in 1984. It was years before I could say the word, "Duchenne" without tears. I wanted to know what my boys were thinking, if they were scared and if they worried about the future, a future that sounded terrifying. I worried but I could not ask. At the same time, I often had the feeling that my sons were protecting me.

What if you could look at Duchenne through your son's eyes? It is a risk, but if even for one moment you could see a different side of things it just might help you, help your son and help everyone you know. You will find your son is quite strong, stronger than you ever guessed. You will learn about his interests, his wishes, and his hope. And you will smile.

Josh Winheld has opened a window. He has chosen to live, and live well. And thankfully, Josh has invited us into his world to learn, to laugh and to enjoy.

Writing the Foreword for this book has been an honor. Josh is a wonderful teacher, and I am a thankful student.

Pat Furlong, President
Parent Project Muscular Dystrophy
www.parentprojectmd.org

Parent Project Muscular Dystrophy is a not-for-profit organization founded in 1994 by parents of children with Duchenne and Becker muscular dystrophy. This organization is dedicated to helping improve the treatment, quality of life, and outlook for the individuals affected by this disease.

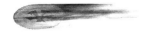

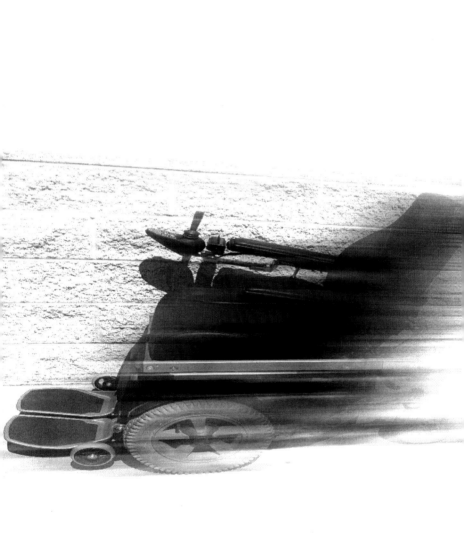

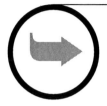

I was starving to death. Breathing was a struggle. My heart was racing all the time. I needed a tracheostomy and a feeding tube or I was going to die.

The choice seemed obvious at the time. I had a thesis to write and a master's degree to complete. I was going to be an urban planner making Philadelphia, my favorite city in the world, a better place to live. I consented to the surgery, figuring it would be a speed bump in life from which I would move on.

The fact that I have Duchenne muscular dystrophy, which causes the muscles in my body to waste away, robbed me of the ability to walk when I was a child, and would one day kill me, never stopped me from accomplishing anything. Why would things be any different this time?

Yet, when I did not finish my thesis or complete my

master's degree I began to question my decision to have the surgery. What was the point of being alive if I was not doing anything productive with my life? I was not ready to give up, but had absolutely no idea what I was going to do.

This book is my answer to that question. In a sense, it is the thesis I never wrote. Only instead of writing about cities, I have written about something far more personal.

I contemplated writing a book for several years. After undergoing surgery nearly three years after my tracheotomy to implant a defibrillator that would protect me from potentially fatal heart rhythms, I knew it was time. After all, if I went through much more I might run out of space to write!

On a serious note I realized just how tenuous my hold on life was. For so long, I had been ahead of the curve in terms of the progression of my disease. Now my heart, the single largest concern for anyone with my disease, was in bad shape. I was running out of time.

Lucky to be alive in the first place, I knew others with my disease who had not been so fortunate. I could have died when working too hard and starving myself in college, or could have been stopped cold by a fatal heart rhythm before deciding to get a defibrillator.

Writing a book takes time. I have been told that completing it in little more than a year is quite an accomplishment. Not having the luxury of time and driven by an almost constant fear that I might not live long enough to finish it, my wish is to see the day it is published. I certainly don't want someone else going out and promoting my book. After all, I am much better looking in person!

Having decided to embark on this project, I knew it would be important to discuss even the most serious, embarrassing aspects of my life. That meant writing about bowel problems and addressing sexuality and death, topics I would ordinarily never talk about with anyone. I have strived to maintain a sense of humor, as many of the serious situations throughout my journey included some downright funny moments even if I didn't think so at the time. In some cases, not choosing to laugh I would have cried and I much prefer to laugh.

Personally speaking, writing this book has allowed me to reflect on my life in a way that I might not have otherwise done. It has given me a greater appreciation for the opportunities presented to me, and a chance to relive moments in my life, both good and bad, that have shaped the person I am today. It has also given me the opportunity to reconnect with many people with whom I had fallen out of touch.

This book is not just about me; I truly believe it is just as much the story of anyone who has lived with this disease. Although my circumstances may be different from another person living with Duchenne muscular dystrophy, there are undoubtedly many experiences we have in common.

I always felt that if I had to have this disease, some good ought to come from it. To that end it's my sincere wish that my story will add to the wealth of knowledge that exists on living with serious illnesses, and includes stories about people with paralysis, cancer, ALS and mental illness, among others.

Hopefully it will offer doctors, nurses, social workers and other professionals who treat people with Duchenne insight on what living with the disease is like for patients and their families, from their day-to-day experiences to a wide range of emotions they may face.

More importantly, it's my wish that my story serves as a source of encouragement to other people with the disease and their families, particularly those who have recently received a diagnosis of Duchenne. Such a diagnosis need not be viewed as the end of the world. It may not always be easy, but life can still be good.

Certainly, everyone hopes for a cure. Perhaps those newly diagnosed will see that day. Older patients like me are unlikely to be around when that day comes, although our lives have been extended with the advent of spinal fusion and ventilators. Sharing my story will be a success if it encourages other patients and their families to live for today, as there is so much they can do.

I may not have a career improving cities or raise a family, but if writing this book is the only thing I ever do, I can live with that. Muscular dystrophy can take away just about everything, but through the written word it can never take away my voice!

~Josh Winheld

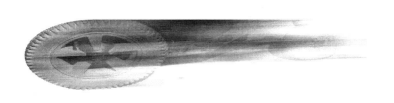

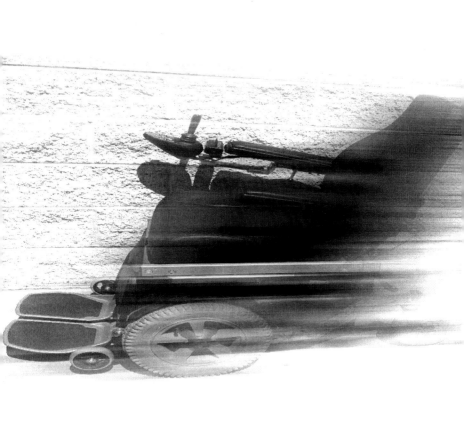

The Diagnosis

1

I couldn't understand why Mom was waking me up in the middle of the night, saying something about going for a ride.

It's still dark outside. How could it be morning already!

Mom helped me get dressed and walked me out to the car; she was not feeling well that day, so it was just going to be Dad and me. I didn't mind because this meant I got to sit up front.

Barely awake as we rode on that late October morning, I was mesmerized by the bright traffic lights and surprised by how few cars were on the streets at that hour. I wondered where we were going.

There was no way Dad could have explained that I would soon undergo a muscle biopsy to confirm that I had a deadly disease that would eventually rob me of the ability to walk, attack my heart and lungs, and kill me by my late teens. This was difficult for any *parent* to comprehend, much less a four-year-old child.

Shortly after arriving at the hospital, a nurse came to take me away. My birth had been one of the best moments in Dad's life...this was one of the worst. But I had no idea. Walking with the nurse, I turned back and smiled. After I was gone, Dad wept quietly for several minutes before regaining composure.

Not long thereafter, the nurse returned to tell him that the procedure was over. She explained that the piece of muscle removed from my thigh had definitely looked diseased. And so Dad cried again.

I awoke in the recovery area in a hospital bed with the rails raised.

Why am I in a crib? I'm not a baby!

The next thing I remember was being pushed to the car in a wheelchair by a nurse. Dad was relieved that although groggy, I was still "happy go lucky." The nurse helped me into the vehicle, handing me a plastic dish in case the anesthesia caused me to throw up.

Once home, I lay down on the sofa where my attentive little sister covered me with a blanket. I stayed home from preschool for several days while recuperating. My classmates painted pictures that were stapled into a get-well booklet.

Each night in the bathtub, I soaked the bandage covering the inch-long horizontal incision on my left thigh; it looked like a great big Band-Aid. I played with syringes the nurses gave me at the hospital, filling them with water and squirting the bathroom walls.

Meanwhile, my parents waited for the conclusive results of the biopsy. Soon they learned just how different their young son's life would be from what they had envisioned.

———————●———————

The afternoon before my birth was snowy with a heavy accumulation predicted overnight in the Philadelphia area. Naturally, that was when Mom decided it was time to go to the hospital!

I was born shortly before 2 A.M. on March 4, 1978, a healthy baby boy from all appearances. Early that morning, my proud dad began calling family and friends with the big news. After finding his car, no easy task in the snow-covered parking lot, he helped the manager of Baby Towne open the store where he bought the biggest stuffed animal he could find.

By all accounts, I was a happy, content baby. I slept well, especially when Mom pushed me for long walks in the stroller. When my aunt came to babysit hoping to play with her nephew, I slept the entire time. After getting a bath, I enjoyed being dried by Dad, who practically polished me like a bowling ball.

I was extremely talkative, making up my own words for anything from foods to family members' names. Although easy-going, I liked options. While it seemed I was having fun spending the night with my aunt when my parents were out of town, out of the blue I would announce that I was "ready to go home now."

My parents and relatives were convinced I was an intelligent child. I loved books and my favorite thing to do was working on puzzles, often turning the pieces over and putting them together without pictures to guide me. I was someone with whom an adult could hold a conversation. An observant child, I easily fixated on objects like bridges pointing out each one and asking lots of questions, sometimes to the point of driving my family insane. "How come we're not moving, Pop-Pop?" I innocently asked my flustered grandfather one day when his car stalled. He wanted to strangle me!

The first child in the family, I received much attention. Not yet parents, my aunts and uncles fussed over me. My grandparents doted on me, taking me out or inviting me to sleep over. I loved going to my maternal grandparents' where my grandfather and I watched HBO movies. My grandmother baked cookies with me using prepared dough from the store, but to me they were the greatest thing in the world.

I enjoyed outings with my paternal grandparents, fondly recalling taking the train into Center City and shopping at Reading Terminal Market. My step-grandfather, who married into the family not long before I was born, built a model railroad set for me and helped me assemble toys.

I also spent lots of time with my great-grandparents

who lived until I was in college and loved visiting them at their apartment where I would push the elevator buttons and raid their candy jars.

The attention from my family was great, but I also had plenty of friends to keep me occupied. Most of them lived on the modest Northeast Philadelphia block of row homes where we lived during my early childhood. Enrolled in preschool at a nearby synagogue, I made friends easily and went on play dates at their homes.

With the birth of my sister Amy when I was three years old, I had a new companion. My affection for her was not immediately obvious. "I don't want that one, I want a different one," I complained when Dad pointed out my baby sister through the nursery window at the hospital. However, it wasn't long before I wanted nothing more than to be her best friend and was disappointed when she wasn't interested in playing. I embraced my role as big brother, and took pride in showing her the way with each stage of life, from preschool to college.

Because there was another child and I was nearing school age, my parents bought a home in nearby Cheltenham Township where they had grown up. It offered an excellent public school system. The three bedroom brick colonial was just down the street from the elementary school and minutes away from both sets of grandparents. It was across the street from a golf course, and I started collecting the multi-colored, dimpled balls that landed on our front lawn.

Not long after we moved in, my parents received the worst news any parents could receive about their child.

While my intellectual and social growth had been quite normal, my parents were concerned fairly early on that my physical development seemed unusually slow. I was unable to sit up by myself as soon as most babies and didn't begin to walk until later than other children. When I finally did, it appeared that my gait waddled. Getting up from the floor was difficult; Mom had to teach me how to walk up steps and spent hours helping me ride my tricycle.

"All kids develop at their own pace," my parents were assured by my first pediatrician. They just needed to continue being supportive parents and everything would be fine, but my parents were not so sure. It seemed obvious that there was something unusual about me. Family members noticed as well, though some were more vocal than others.

My parents took me to several orthopedic specialists, all of whom seemed "basically clueless," according to Mom. After watching me walk, one doctor told my parents, "I walked like that when I was a kid and I turned out just fine."

Finally, they took me to another pediatrician. After observing my unusual gait when I walked into the examining room, he noticed that my calves seemed overdeveloped for my age. He asked me to sit down on the floor and then asked me to get up without holding onto anything. The only way I could do this was by getting on my hands and knees, then using my hands to climb up my legs and thighs.

These were classic symptoms of muscular dystrophy. Throughout thirty years in private practice the doctor had never seen a child with muscular dystrophy, but when he examined me, a bell went off in his head.

Although he was virtually certain of the diagnosis, he simply told my parents, "This is what it could be..." and sent us to a doctor at a nearby hospital who ordered a blood test called a CPK, short for creatine phosphokinase. A very high level in the blood was an indicator of the type of muscle breakdown associated with muscular dystrophy.

"There are 40 different neuromuscular diseases and I believe Josh has one of them," the doctor told my parents before the blood test was performed. "But I don't think it is one that we need to be worried about."

When the test results came in off the charts, the doctor changed his tune in a hurry. Now there was good reason to be worried, and he referred us to The Children's Hospital of Philadelphia (CHOP) which had greater expertise in neuromuscular diseases.

We met for the first time with the neurologist who would follow me for the next fifteen years. The doctor, a muscular dystrophy researcher at the University of Pennsylvania, was about my parents' age. He stood tall, wore a beard, and was soft-spoken with a professorial demeanor and a disarming presence about him.

That was until he reached into his doctor's bag and pulled out a yellow rubber tourniquet and a syringe to collect a blood sample for a repeat CPK test. I clung to my mom as if she would somehow protect me, but this was one time she couldn't. I screamed like any other child scared at the sight of a needle. The doctor told my parents he had a son my age and grinned as if to say, "Come on kid, don't make me feel any worse about this than I already do."

Although having the blood drawn was not nearly as bad as I anticipated, going to checkups for the next several years brought with it the apprehension of having blood drawn.

The test results were just as alarming as the first test. A normal CPK level was 235 or below, mine was more than 10,000! Muscle breakdown was clearly occurring and Duchenne, a serious and life-threatening form of muscular dystrophy, was most likely the cause.

To measure changes in electrical activity within muscle, which is another indicator of the disease, the doctor ordered a test called an EMG, or electromyography. Considering how much fun the CPK test had been, the EMG during which electrodes were inserted into various muscles while small electrical impulses were delivered was no less frightening. The EMG results also indicated an abnormality in my muscles.

The last test to confirm a diagnosis of Duchenne muscular dystrophy was the muscle biopsy, the thought of which was heart-breaking for my parents. Still, it would offer a definitive explanation for the physical difficulties I was experiencing.

Once the results of the muscle biopsy were available, my parents met with the neurologist who explained the findings. As predicted, I had Duchenne muscular dystrophy, a disorder that causes progressive muscle wasting and weakening primarily in the skeletal muscles of the body and in the heart and muscles used for breathing. In some cases, though not mine, it even causes learning disabilities. The disorder nearly always affects boys and is the result of a mutation on the x chromosome inherited from their moms who usually have no symptoms.

The prognosis was bleak. By age 10 most patients needed wheelchairs and at the time most died by their late teens. There was no treatment or cure for the disease, with its cause essentially unknown at that point. Other than the promise of ongoing research and the fact that I was still young, there was not much hope the doctor could offer.

As they sat there listening to the doctor, my parents didn't cry or hold each other; they basically already knew what the results meant. Still, it was devastating news. Their son had been given a death sentence and there was nothing they could do, no way to fix the problem.

In the weeks that followed, my parents went through periods of grief, fear and depression. Mom did her best to stay busy, seeing little point in dwelling on the bad news. Dad talked to a rabbi, but didn't find much comfort. Neither of my parents spent much time asking why. "It didn't change the past and it doesn't change the future," Dad felt.

Family members and friends were kept in the loop from the beginning, and my parents leaned on them for support. My maternal grandmother who was battling breast cancer at the time took the news hard but was a major source of comfort for Mom, as was one of my aunts. Another aunt and uncle researched everything they could about the disease. Everyone was truly upset for my parents and for me.

Getting involved with a support group for parents of local boys with Duchenne was especially helpful for Mom and Dad. Through the group, they were able to learn what to expect down the road from parents of children a few years older than I was.

They went on with life hopeful that a treatment might be found, never looking too far into the future, taking the progression of the disease as it came. To stay abreast of the latest research developments, my parents asked plenty of questions when we went to the muscular dystrophy clinic at the hospital for my checkups. They became involved with the Muscular Dystrophy Association (MDA). Every Labor Day, Dad and a few family members volunteered at the local broadcast of the Jerry Lewis MDA Telethon. When my sister and I were older, we too volunteered. The free food was a wonderful perk!

Other than making sure I was seen regularly at the muscular dystrophy clinic, there was not a whole lot my parents could do from a medical standpoint. Still, they tried to help me strengthen my muscles, purchasing one -pound weights for me to use. My neurologist told them that limited exercise could be beneficial, though too much could accelerate the muscle breakdown process.

They also took me to a doctor specializing in vitamin therapy. I liked this doctor because he didn't draw any blood. All the information he needed could be obtained by analyzing a single strand of my hair. But I did not enjoy taking the vitamins he prescribed. I hadn't learned to swallow pills yet, so I had to take the foul-tasting chewable versions.

Whether any of this helped was unclear, but my parents felt they were at least doing something.

Somehow, during these early years my parents told me about my disease, my "problem" as we referred to it, though there was no single specific conversation that I can recall. At the dinner table one evening shortly after my diagnosis, I listened as Dad explained to my sister why I fell down so often and couldn't run as fast as other kids.

By then, everything he said was already familiar to me and not a big deal. Maybe it wasn't easy getting up from the floor or walking up stairs, but I could still do it. Sometimes it hurt when I fell, but then I got up and was fine. I wasn't sick. I just had a problem.

In time, I learned more about my "problem" and its ultimate outcome. But there would be time for that later, much, much later, my parents hoped and prayed.

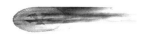

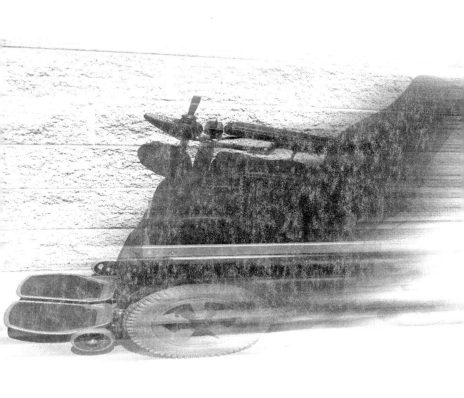

2

After learning of my diag-
nosis the previous year, my parents made the decision
not to place me in an alternative school. The muscles in
my body may have been deteriorating, but there was
clearly nothing wrong with my mind. Nor did I have any
significant physical limitations that would prevent me
from attending a regular school. My parents met with
the principal before I entered kindergarten, informing
him of my disease and making it clear that I was to be
treated like any other student.

Once school began, I adjusted with no difficulty. I
made friends easily, followed the rules, and paid attention during lessons. I was self-motivated, enjoying any
opportunity to learn something new. My good memory helped, in that I could easily retain facts, dates, and
spelling lists. Learning to read opened up a whole new
world and I would read anything I could get my hands

on, including any bills or documents sitting on Mom's kitchen desk!

My favorite subject in school was history; I enjoyed lessons about figures like Abraham Lincoln and events like the signing of the Declaration of Independence.

Math however, did not come easily. Mastering subtraction proved especially frustrating, with many tears shed over homework assignments on the subject. Long division was not much easier. My teacher wrote a note at the bottom of a returned test, stating that I was a smart kid even if I tried to "change the rules pertaining to long division!"

Though my teachers saw me as a bright child I never felt especially intelligent, lacking in self-confidence, afraid to make mistakes and raising my hand only when sure of the answer. I cringed when the teacher called on me out of the blue.

Away from the classroom I looked forward to special activities during the course of the school day, whether it was the chance to be creative in art, sing along to the piano in music, or choose books to take out of the school library. I even liked the games and exercises in gym, although I developed an early fear of basketball. I could throw the ball toward the net, but when it inevitably missed I wasn't coordinated enough to move out of the way fast enough to avoid getting clunked in the head!

When it was time for recess, I couldn't wait to get outside in the fresh air and run around, wind in my face. I felt the strain in my weakened legs as I struggled to walk with my hands on my thighs, up the steep hill connecting the parking lot to the playing field below. In the fall, I loved to run down a small embankment into a huge pile of leaves against the fence.

As much as I enjoyed school, there were times when being the only physically disabled child proved difficult. I often struggled to keep up with the other kids, unable to get up from the floor as quickly or run as fast at recess. Putting on a heavy coat, a simple task for everyone else required every bit of coordination I could muster. I moved about in a deliberate, cautious manner, in constant fear of being inadvertently knocked down by children in the hallway.

While I never felt ashamed of my "problem," other students' reaction to the attention I received on account of it was quite upsetting. Some thought I was merely looking for attention when I suddenly fell. Classmates became jealous when teachers allowed me to sit on a chair instead of the floor with everyone else because I was having trouble getting up from the floor. "Why does Josh get to sit in a chair?" they asked. My face turned beet red and I remember wishing that I could disappear. The last thing I wanted was to be different from everyone else.

I want to sit on the floor just like you.

From that moment on, I always felt uncomfortable when teachers paid extra attention to me on account of my disability for fear that others would be envious or that they would think I was a teacher's pet. For many years, I constantly worried that my classmates would look at any academic recognition I received as the result of teachers' feeling sorry for me.

During recess I endured the cruel taunts, teases and occasional shoves and pushes from kids, sometimes even from my friends who noticed that I walked and ran differently or like a "cripple" or "retard," as they told me. Sometimes they imitated how I walked.

Their actions and words often reduced me to tears, as much as I tried to avoid crying in front of them. "I do not walk like that!" I insisted, convinced they had it all wrong.

I have a problem, but there's nothing wrong with the way I walk!

When I came home, Mom listened sympathetically and tried to comfort me as I sobbed through my account of the day's events. On the other hand, Dad encouraged me to respond to my tormentors by calling them names. Unfortunately, I wasn't especially creative when it came to name-calling.

The day did come however, when I reached my boiling point. Provoked at lunch by a big burly kid who had been picking on me for weeks, I rose up from my seat, stretched across the table, grabbed his milk carton, and poured it all over the food on his lunch tray. I felt an incredible sense of satisfaction until, of course he responded in kind. I burst into tears, and both of us were sent to the principal's office!

As I waited on the bench outside the office for the principal to emerge, I trembled with fear. I had never been sent to the principal's office before. That was only for the bad kids. Still, I felt my actions were justified.

Through tears, I told my side of the story to the principal, a tall, bald, stern-looking man who addressed students gathered at assemblies like a drill sergeant. In the end, I got off with a warning after promising to never take matters into my own hands like that again.

To help me deal with my fears and frustrations, arrangements were made for me to see the school psychologist on a weekly basis, which allowed me to get things off my chest. What I mostly enjoyed about this was missing class time to talk about my day-to-day experiences with an adult who was willing to listen.

After all, it wasn't as if my life outside of school was unusual in any way. My parents provided a stable, comfortable lifestyle for my sister and me. Mom stayed at home with us and ran the house with efficiency, keeping everything neat and orderly down to the coupons that she wouldn't be caught dead without at the supermarket.

She picked out our clothes in the morning, packed a nutritious lunch, and made sure homework was completed right after school. A well-balanced meal was on the table practically every night, and bedtime was strictly enforced. I was not allowed to stay up to watch the TV shows that everyone was talking about in school. Mom played board games with us (always letting us win), baked cookies with us, and even sewed Halloween costumes. One year we were Crayola Crayons, yellow for me, pink for Amy.

Dad kept regular hours at his insurance agency and was home nearly every night with us. When my sister or I had a special event, he never missed it. The disciplinarian of the house right down to table manners, he also had a fun, juvenile side, playing Wiffle ball and Frisbee in the yard with us and enjoying a good practical joke. Time and time again, he tricked me with the supposedly faulty garden hose.

"Come over here for a second. I can't get this thing to work," he told me. When I approached, he turned it on full throttle, completely soaking my clothes. I ran away but kept coming back for more.

"Get Amy, too!" I encouraged him, but my sister was not nearly as gullible.

We spent plenty of time together, especially playing in the backyard where Dad had installed a swing set. In my first couple of years of school, I was so excited about what I learned that I held "school" and tried to teach Amy, then in preschool and not especially interested in my lessons. Various activities kept me fairly busy; I took art classes at the community center and piano lessons through my granddad's music school. Although I had some difficulty attaining the proper hand posture, my greatest problem was that I hated to practice.

Sunday mornings found me in religious school, where I enjoyed learning about the Jewish holidays. In the summer, I attended day camp, struggling at times to keep up with other children but not enough to affect my overall experience.

For obvious reasons I did not participate in any athletic activities during the school year, and didn't like sports anyway. Afraid of getting hurt, I didn't envy my friends in that regard. But it made getting together with them on Saturday mornings difficult because they were all busy.

I moved at a slower pace than other children, but was relatively active. Jumping in leaves, sledding in the snow, and swimming at the local pool were some of the outdoor activities I enjoyed in addition to playing with other children my age, inviting them over or going to their houses. My friends' parents were all somehow aware that I was different from other kids although my parents told few, if any of them. They did not keep my disease a secret, but the subject didn't often come up.

Perhaps this was because at the time my disease did not make me look a whole lot different from other children. Other than my enlarged, muscular-looking calves, I certainly didn't look different except for my unsteady gait, walking on my toes with my belly sticking out in order to balance myself. I did have a propensity to stumble and fall, and walking up and down steps was difficult. I tired more easily with physical activity.

There was not much maintenance required to manage my disease. After walking long distances or otherwise over-exerting myself, I smeared on smelly sports rubs and used a heating pad to relieve painful cramps in the back of my legs. I wore splints every night — we called them "night shoes"— to keep my ankles and feet straight. They were really no big deal except when I had to get out of bed in the middle of the night to go to the bathroom. But I would say anything to con my neighbor out of making me wear them when she babysat.

"I don't have to wear them tonight. Mom and Dad said so," I told her.

"Are you *sure* that's what they said?" she asked.

"Sometimes they let me skip them," I insisted.

"Okay, but I better not get in trouble for this," she warned.

I learned my limitations and managed to adapt without even realizing it. I was cautious when someplace unfamiliar, and was hesitant to move quickly on uneven surfaces. I resorted to crawling up the steps and sliding down them on my butt. It was safer and more efficient. I didn't spend time thinking about the fact that I had to do things differently. My habits became ingrained and unworthy of a second thought.

It helped that my parents treated whatever issues that arose with a matter-of-fact attitude. When I fell down, I often got upset but got over it quickly because they never made a big deal about it.

I remember falling face-first on the hardwood floor in the dining room, knocking out at least one of my top front baby teeth. Hearing me shriek, Dad came quickly from the other room. I wasn't seriously hurt, so he simply helped me to my feet, issued his patented "You're okay," got me some ice, and that was the end of it.

Of course, Mom was somewhat horrified to return

home to find me with a big gap between my front teeth! "How did *that* happen?" she asked Dad.

"He's *fine,*" he said.

Dad often tried to use his sense of humor to make me feel better. When I came home from school and was upset that I had fallen three times that day, he reminded me that it was better than falling down four times the previous day.

It also helped to know that I was not the only one with physical problems. Mom told me about conversations she had with my grandmother, then with late-stage cancer. "Mom-mom is having trouble walking up steps too, you know," she told me.

My parents never babied me. There was never the sense of, "Oh, look at poor Josh. He's sick and going to die. We need to make things easier for him." The last thing they wanted was for me to use my disability as an excuse. They always made me do whatever I could for myself. Even if I was tired, I had to walk up the steps. If something was out of my reach, I had to get up and get it for myself. Just because something wasn't easy for me didn't mean I shouldn't do it for myself.

With my sister in the picture, I realized early on that the world did not revolve around me. To the best of their ability, my parents tried to make sure that I was not always the center of their attention. Amy's ballet recitals were always a big deal in our house. I needed more help, but my sister deserved equal attention. Naturally, she grew jealous of me anyway but I never received the impression that my needs were more important than hers even if I sometimes wished they were.

I certainly never felt that I could misbehave and get away with it because my parents felt sorry for me. Cautious and afraid of falling, I never had to be corrected for climbing on furniture or for being too wild around the house. But I picked on my sister. And I got in trouble with my mouth. Around other adults, I was always on my best behavior. With my parents, I talked back and developed a reputation for always getting in the last word.

Disease or no disease my parents punished me, whether it meant scolding me, taking away certain privileges, sending me to my bedroom, or even spanking me on a rare occasion.

Still, it wasn't as if I didn't get any positive attention on account of my disease. When I was eight years old, I was chosen as poster child for the southeastern Pennsylvania chapter of the Muscular Dystrophy Association (MDA). Dad had become friendly with one of the MDA coordinators through his annual volunteer work for the local broadcast of the Jerry Lewis Telethon, who asked whether I might be interested in being considered for the position of poster child.

It sounded like fun to me. After being officially selected, I began a whirlwind tour of fundraisers, interviews, and appearances with local celebrities and dignitaries like the mayor of Philadelphia. I attended dance marathons at local universities, golf outings, store openings, concerts, and business gatherings — anything to raise funds for MDA and to create awareness about muscular dystrophy.

The attention was wonderful. For an eight-year-old, there was nothing better than collecting a vast array of logo-adorned shirts, hats, pens, key-chains and photos, posters and autographs. But there were also some rather unique opportunities. I was featured in a segment during the telethon broadcast, read the weather report on a local rock station, and rode in the "cherry-picker" of a Philadelphia fire truck.

We attended a number of the events as a family and the event coordinators tried to make my sister feel included; she was right there with me in the cherry-picker, but more often it was just me and Dad. Not only was this a great father-son bonding opportunity, but Dad took a lot of pressure off of me with his outgoing personality that made him comfortable engaging in conversation.

It turned out to be a special time to be poster child. That year, scientists identified the gene that mutated to cause Duchenne. Looking to put a face to the disease, all three local TV stations converged on our home. They filmed me playing the piano, walking down the steps at home, and interacting with my sister. I enjoyed being on camera, but was mortified that one crew shot me walking outside when I suddenly fell and began to cry.

The missing protein associated with the gene called "dystrophin" was identified the following year, and the media descended upon us again.

My work as poster child helped to foster awareness and understanding of my disease at school. Who else could have brought in a tape of himself reading the weather on the radio or wearing an Honorary Fire Chief helmet to show-and-tell? With the teacher's help I talked to my classmates about my disease, explaining why I walked differently and fell so much. I even brought in my "night shoes" to show the class, and developed a sense of pride about being different.

It could not have come at a better time. By then my disease was starting to really affect me. I was having much more difficulty walking and I fell more often. I became particularly afraid of falling down stairs, and walked almost sideways holding onto the railing with both hands. I stopped going to gym, unable to keep up with the other kids.

As my classmates became more aware of my disease, they were more willing to help me. One of my close friends made sure to hold on to my arm as we walked downstairs to the cafeteria. Of course, helping me came with the added benefit of being first in the lunch line because the teacher let us leave a few minutes before everyone else to avoid crowds.

I also became more aware of my disease and how it would affect my future. At the MDA events I attended as poster child, I met some of the older boys with Duchenne who were already in motorized wheelchairs so it became apparent that I would eventually need a wheelchair, too. But it didn't seem so bad.

It looks like fun — and I won't have to walk and get so tired.

One day, while searching for toilet reading material, I found a few MDA pamphlets about Duchenne and decided to read them in the privacy of the bathroom. When I first read what one pamphlet said about life expectancy, it sounded scary. Then I thought about it.

How could I die? I feel perfectly fine. That's not going to happen to me.

The only experience I had with death was when my grandmother died of cancer. Before she died, she looked thin and frail and always seemed to be asleep on the sofa, bundled in blankets.

I was nothing like that. Even if I was going to die, it wasn't going to happen for a long time. I never told my parents about what I had read, figuring they had chosen not to tell me so I wouldn't be scared. Besides, I was not sure if I was supposed to have read the pamphlets and didn't want to get in trouble.

Mom and Dad were more concerned about the immediate future. With my ability to walk steadily declining, they began searching for a house that could accommodate a wheelchair. Aware of their search, I began excitedly pointing out ranch houses whenever we drove anywhere.

I'll never have to walk up steps to get to my room!

Of course, my parents were just a bit more selective than I. They hoped to find a suitable home in the same township and preferably within the boundaries of our current elementary school, so my sister and I could remain in the same school district.

In the spring of 1986, they bought a home practically a stone's throw from where we currently lived. Nearly all of my friends lived in the neighborhood, so I was thrilled.

Naturally, I managed to fall and skin my knee the first time I visited the house, but once the bleeding stopped and I wiped the tears from my eyes I liked what I saw. The bedroom that was to be mine was on the first floor; it had three windows and a bathroom next door. There was a huge backyard behind the house. And because the previous owner had been disabled, the house had grab bars in the bathroom, a door-buzzer system, and a stair glide to reach the basement.

Once we moved in, all kinds of renovations began. The kitchen was completely overhauled, the large picture window removed and replaced with sliding glass doors that opened onto a deck that was being added. Instead of steps, a long ramp down to the backyard was constructed to accommodate a wheelchair. The garage was converted into a large family room and the floor was raised so it would be level with the rest of the house.

The next summer I attended a week-long overnight camp designed for children with muscular dystrophy. Still able to walk, I had a chance to watch the boys who were in motorized wheelchairs full-time, and to learn how they carried out their daily activities of getting dressed, transferring in and out of their chairs, going to the bathroom, and bathing. I saw what happened when their wheelchairs malfunctioned. Most of all, I noticed how dignified they were despite their limitations and the help they required. I was amazed at how calm they were when things didn't go exactly right. And I saw how they still managed to do as much as the campers who could walk.

The camp truly pushed the envelope. Held at a Boy Scout camp in the New Jersey Pine Barrens that my great-uncle had attended back in the Stone Ages, it didn't seem that the rustic facilities had changed much since then. The cabins were square shacks with screens on three sides and bunk beds mounted on the walls. Bathroom and shower facilities were located across the camp.

When it rained, which it did most of the week, the paths became muddy and impossible for a wheelchair to navigate through. Sheets of plywood had to be laid out across the camp. The next summer, a permanent "board-walk" was constructed on the grounds.

A few buildings had electricity, one where motorized wheelchairs were taken at night for charging, which the counselors loved because it gave them a chance to race each other. Of course not having a wheelchair nearby had its drawbacks, particularly when one of my bunk-mates had a late night upset stomach. His counselor had no other option but to scoop him out of bed and race to the nearest bathroom. I don't remember if they made it in time!

The activities at the camp were the same as at a camp for children without disabilities and included swimming in the lake, canoeing, fishing, horseback riding, archery and rocketry, albeit with assistance. There was no thought of arranging alternative activities because campers were "fragile."

The counselors, all volunteers, were practically teenagers and assigned one-on-one to campers. As I was among the younger male campers and since there were more female volunteers, I was matched with a pretty blonde the first year. Dad was impressed, even if I wasn't.

A girl? Why couldn't I have gotten a cool guy instead?

I doubted I would have as much fun with a female assistant. As it turned out, the bigger concern was being seen naked in front of a girl. What was I thinking? Fortunately, I could still dress myself so I was able to have her look the other way while I did that. Showering was a different story. It didn't help that the showers were exceptionally gross, but I wasn't able to regulate the water temperature by myself, and needed some assistance getting washed. You guessed it ... I didn't shower for the entire week!

Although it was my first time away from home for an extended period, I had so much fun that I wasn't the least bit homesick. There was something to do practically every second. I enjoyed the nighttime activities that were based on each year's theme. I loved the silly events that took place during the course of the day, from harassing kitchen staff to get them to let us in the dining hall, to hanging underwear on the flagpole.

When my parents and sister came to pick me up at the end of the week, I gushed with excitement as I told them about the fun I had. They had some exciting news to share as well; Mom was pregnant.

I was ecstatic, having often thought about what it might be like to have another sibling; it seemed like it would be fun. I couldn't wait to help pick out a name.

For my parents, there were greater concerns. If the baby turned out to be a boy, there was a 50 percent chance that he would have Duchenne, as Mom was a carrier of the disease. At the time, there was no way to test a fetus for the disease, but she was able to undergo a relatively new procedure that could determine the sex of the baby earlier than had been possible before and could also identify certain other serious genetic disorders. If it was determined that the fetus was male, my parents would have faced a tough decision. Much to their relief the test results revealed that the baby was female, and they prepared to welcome another daughter into the world.

Meanwhile Mom and Dad continued to prepare for the time when I would be wheelchair-dependent, purchasing a brown Chevrolet minivan that they would eventually have converted to accommodate a wheelchair. The day Dad picked the van up at the dealership turned out to be the day that my paternal grandfather died in the hospital after a long battle with heart disease. When he returned home that evening with the van, he looked drained. I was not sure what to say. Though I had not been very close with my grandfather, I understood the significance for my dad. "Sorry about your dad," I said to him when he came home, and even in light of what had happened he still took me for a ride around the neighborhood in the new van, a tradition whenever he brought home a new car.

The next day I accompanied him to my grandfather's house in New Jersey, where family and friends were gathering. On the ride home, few words were spoken as we listened to Phil Collins on the tape deck, but I loved being with my dad at that moment. He was so protective, making sure I wasn't too cold and putting his arm in front of me when he stopped short at a traffic light. If only he could have protected me from the inevitable path of my disease.

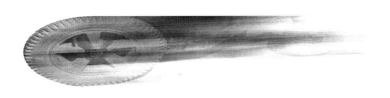

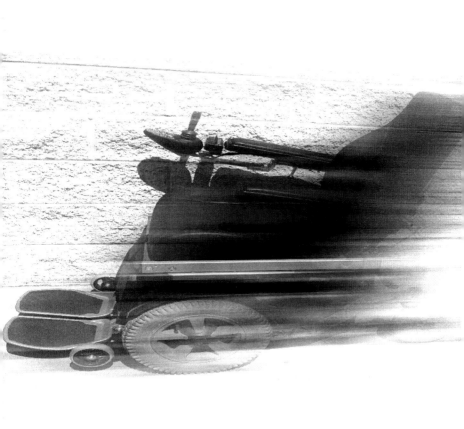

When my first motorized wheelchair arrived the summer before I entered fourth grade, my parents promptly stuck it in the corner of the dining room. While my ability to walk had been steadily declining, the plan was for me to keep walking as long as possible. They understood that the more I used the wheelchair, the more dependent I would become, and didn't want to encourage me to use it until absolutely necessary.

At that time, the wheelchair came with a staggering $4,000 price tag, fortunately covered by insurance. It was basically a manual wheelchair with a motor box mounted just above the rear wheels, and was powered by two car batteries beneath the padded blue vinyl seat and operated by moving a video game-style joystick. It even had a horn!

By the time school started that fall, it was abundantly clear that the time had arrived for me to start using the wheelchair. I was increasingly unsteady on my feet especially on the plush carpeting in the house, often holding on to the newly painted white walls, at times even resorting to crawling to the nearest piece of furniture to pull myself up.

My legs were so tired from supporting my body that I was in constant fear they would give out at any second, and was always glad when I fell on carpet or grass although I wasn't always so lucky. Even when I did not fall, walking was an exhausting proposition and I avoided moving around more than necessary.

Initially, I got out of my wheelchair frequently to sit on the sofa or floor at home or at my desk when I was in school. During the next several months however, I grew weaker and transferred out of the wheelchair less and less.

Being in a wheelchair was not at all devastating; in fact I barely gave it a second thought, simply accepting the situation for what it was. I wasn't able to walk anymore and needed it to go about my daily routine. I was too young to fully grasp the idea that this was the first major change the disease caused in my life. My parents certainly never made a big deal about it in front of me.

I wasn't angry or upset that I could no longer walk like everyone else. I wasn't ashamed of my body, if anything a tremendous sense of relief came over me. I would no longer have to worry about sudden falls, and could go as far as the other kids without getting tired or struggling to walk as quickly. I actually looked and felt more normal in a wheelchair because no one would be able to see that I walked funny, no one would gawk when I fell and started to cry.

Plus, how cool was it that before I was even 10 years old I could "drive?" I loved getting in the chair and buckling up just like in a car, turning on the power, unlocking the brakes, and zooming around the house. I beeped the horn at the cat and laughed as the frightened feline darted down the basement steps. Showing off for family friends was a new-found delight. No, there was nothing bad about the wheelchair!

The first day my new wheels took me to school I had butterflies in my stomach. What would everybody say? Would they make a big deal out of it? It wasn't long before I realized that a motorized wheelchair was a real attention-grabber. Everybody wanted to check out my chair, even the kids who used to pick on me. My teacher wanted to know if it came with air conditioning like the similarly priced Yugo automobile!

Just before class began a crowd formed around me. "How do you drive it?" asked one kid. "How fast can it go?" Someone else insisted that I beep the horn. Pulling up to my desk, I carefully transferred to the seat. "Can I get in?" another kid asked. I tried with no success to tell my peers that I wasn't supposed to let anyone in the wheelchair. The begging continued, "Come on, just for a second." I loved the attention and hated to turn my curious classmates down, but I wasn't about to trust them with my baby. "NO!" I said emphatically, finally ending all discussion.

Even so, my chair continued to gain me attention throughout the year. Outside during recess and in hallways when no adults were looking, I raced my friends. That fall, for the school Halloween parade, we turned it into a military tank by fitting a cardboard box around the chair, attaching an empty paper towel roll for the turret and spray-painting everything green.

The school was well-prepared to accommodate my wheelchair. Prior to the start of the year, my parents and I met with the school district's director of facilities. A pleasant, outgoing man, he gave me a firm handshake and told me that if I encountered any accessibility problems I was to contact him directly. Ramps were installed in a few locations at the school and a stall was widened in the bathroom across from my class. However, the only way for me to reach the cafeteria was to go outside, down a steep driveway. When it was too cold outside, classmates brought my lunch back to the classroom and ate with me.

Always ready to lend a helping hand, my attentive teacher assisted me with tasks like putting on my coat. Classmates were especially protective of me, making sure I didn't fall when transferring from my wheelchair to the desk chair. Each month, I proudly prepared a schedule designating my daily "helper." Each classmate's name appeared at least once, even those I wasn't especially fond of.

Everyone seemed to relish the opportunity to be my

helper for the day. I enjoyed the extra time spent with my friends on those days, even when the pretty girls would lend a helping hand. By then, I was past the "Yuck, girls are gross stage." Still, when I sat alone in the classroom with girls while the teacher was at lunch, a strange tingly sensation rushed over me. I didn't know what it was, but definitely liked the feeling.

The school district provided transportation in a wheelchair-accessible van to get me to and from school. I hated it. The vehicles were old and rickety, and the drivers downright creepy, like the guy who came for me one morning in a late-model powder blue Ford van. He wore a funky-smelling flannel jacket and didn't say two words to me. I backed onto the decrepit lift and hoped it wouldn't get stuck. As he tied my chair down for the short ride to school, the engine sputtered and the smell from the exhaust belched into the air. We started moving, and still not a word from the driver.

"What's your name?" I nervously inquired. "Ray," he mumbled.

"Uh, nice to meet you," I replied. No response. "It's really cold today."

Dead silence engulfed the van. I wondered if there was anything going on inside this man's head or if he was a serial killer in disguise! He sure seemed to fit the profile. I didn't utter another word for the rest of the trip, which seemed to take forever. Never was I happier to arrive at school. Our paths never crossed again, although I always worried that they would.

At home, some adjustments were also necessary. A physical therapist was sent out to evaluate our house and make suggestions. Fortunately, the renovations my parents had made since moving there made it much easier and the bathroom I used was large enough to accommodate my wheelchair. Thanks to the installation of grab bars, I was able to transfer to the toilet independently, though it wouldn't be long before someone would have to lift me. A urinal was also ordered to save me the trouble of getting up every time I had to pee. My face turned beet red. Embarrassed wasn't the word, horrified was more like it. What if everyone at school knew I peed into a bottle? I promptly stuck it in the cabinet beneath the sink

There is no way I'm using that! I can still get up. It's not that big a deal!

Actually, it was a big deal. It was so tiring having to slide my pants down and get out of my chair every time I had to pee. Still, I resisted the temptation to try the urinal. However the afternoon finally came when I really had to go, and making it to the toilet wasn't an option. That was the day I remembered the urinal. Opening the cabinet, I removed the hard blue plastic bottle, its lid marked "URINAL." As if I didn't know. I stared at it for a moment out of morbid curiosity, wondering what it would be like to pee into a bottle. I mean, it certainly wasn't normal. I unzipped my pants, put myself into it and tried to go. I couldn't!

I have to go so bad! Why can't I go? I have to go!

Telling myself it was indeed okay to let it flow even

though I wasn't sitting on the toilet, I finally started to go. It sounded funny as my urine hit the container, which began to feel warm against my leg. Ah, sweet relief! Pretty soon, I couldn't imagine *not* using a urinal. What a difference it made. I could pee as many times a day as I wanted, it was so effortless.

When I had to go to the bathroom at school, I asked a friend to come with me. Entering the accessible stall, I reached into the backpack on my chair for the urinal, relieved myself and emptied it into the toilet. Emerging from the stall, I had my friend rinse it with the liquid soap in my backpack. I double-checked to be sure that the urinal was in the bag and that the bag was zipped. Surprisingly, none of my friends seemed grossed out handling a bottle in which I had just peed. I certainly would have been. But if they were okay with it, so was I.

Back at home, I showered by sitting on a bath seat positioned in range of the water. While transferring to the toilet was still possible, getting into the shower was not so easy. Dad lifted me from the wheelchair to the bath seat. Once he helped me regulate the water temperature, he left the room and closed the door. I could still wash myself thanks to a sponge attached to a plastic handle that was long enough to reach my back and feet. Everything was fine until the toilet was flushed elsewhere in the house. "Daaaaaddd!" I let out a blood-curdling scream as scalding hot water poured over my defenseless body. After that happened a few times, I began avoiding showering as much as possible. Once a week was more than enough!

A few months after transitioning to the wheelchair, our minivan was fully equipped and ready to go. It had a raised roof and a semi-automatic lift, which needed to be manually lowered to floor level. The middle seats were removed to accommodate my wheelchair, which was secured with tie-downs in front and locks in the back that closed when the wheels tripped them.

Even though we had our own vehicle, I continued to use the school district's transportation. Mom was a bit preoccupied with something, rather someone else at the time. My sister Stephanie was born that January. The morning after she was born, Dad woke me to get ready for school. Normally, I preferred when Mom woke me up. She came in quietly, without the light on and gently woke me. Dad was much more abrupt, turning on the light, yanking the covers off, telling me it was time to get up. But when he told me the news, I immediately perked up. Being a big brother again was so exciting; I proudly wore a sweatshirt given to me that identified me as such, though several weeks later I was embarrassed when Mom brought my new sister into school all bundled up for the winter weather wearing a tiny hat and mittens.

Despite being in a wheelchair I still helped take care of my baby sister, supervising her while she played in front of the television watching *Sesame Street*. Sometimes, I found the show more entertaining than she did! I held her in my lap and took turns feeding her when she began eating solid foods.

Eventually, Amy and I babysat for our sister. Though I was growing more limited physically, my parents knew that I was responsible enough to be left in charge. Of course, that didn't stop me from asking Stephanie to hand me the urinal when she was a few years older. Unlike Amy, she was still young enough that she never protested!

Like any older sibling, I became jealous. Stephanie got away with more than Amy and me so we protested even though it was inevitable that my parents would be more laid-back raising their third child. At times, I became frustrated that the attention Mom gave my sister took away from my care.

That summer, I returned to the camp for kids with muscular dystrophy. I also attended a month-long overnight camp for children with all types of disabilities. When we toured the camp the previous summer, I was truly impressed. It looked like a "real" camp facility. The sprawling complex connected by a paved trail contained nearly two dozen fully-accessible cabins with concrete ramps and actual bathrooms inside! There was a large swimming pool, a baseball field, basketball courts, and a field house as well as an indoor pool and gym.

In many ways, it was like any camp for "normal" kids. There were structured activities each day, and evening activities included movies, talent shows and performances by singing groups. There were also special events like dances, field trips, and color wars. The main difference was that most of the campers required assistance from counselors with their daily routines. Each bunk had at least three counselors who would help with bathing, dressing and activities, and to whom campers were expected to address as "Aunt" or "Uncle."

On the one hand, it was nice not to struggle to keep up with the other kids as I had in my years attending day camp. On the other hand, attending a camp with other disabled kids gave me a real appreciation for the fact that I was more normal than many of the other campers.

I learned about other diseases, realizing how fortunate I was. The more seriously disabled campers required complete care. They couldn't speak, their limbs flailed involuntarily and drool constantly rolled down their cheeks. They wore diapers and needed to be fed. Still, many of these campers possessed normal intelligence.

I'm glad I don't have a disease like that. They're like grown babies.

I truly admired some of my bunkmates. There was a blind camper who played in a string band, and another camper with spina bifida whose bowel and bladder function were so impaired that every day he lay down on the cold bathroom floor to catheterize himself and give himself an enema. I was amazed not only at how vigilant he was at his care, but at how he didn't seem the least bit embarrassed when other people walked in and out of the bathroom when he was doing all of this.

As for me, I was horrified at the idea of sitting on the toilet, trying to take a dump while someone else was attempting the same feat on the adjacent throne! After getting washed in the shower, I hated being wheeled out of the bathroom in the shower chair completely naked in front of the rest of the campers.

Of course, that wasn't the most embarrassing thing. Each time someone had a bowel movement, the counselor was supposed to record its size, color and consistency.

"Hey, Uncle Mike! You've got to see this. I've never seen anything quite like it before!"

For many kids camp may have been a great experience. Just not for me. After my first summer, the novelty wore off. Although letters I wrote home indicated that I was having a great time, the reality was that from the second I arrived the countdown to the day it would be over began.

I hated having counselors help me bathe and get dressed. They were too rough, too impatient, and did not like it when I complained. Nor did I enjoy most activities, especially sports. I couldn't play without assistance and could not find any joy in having someone help me shoot a basketball or swing a baseball bat.

It was difficult for me to connect with the other campers. The truth of the matter was that I didn't really like being with other disabled kids. Camp was merely a detour from my normal life. I did not feel like I was one of them. Nothing that happened at camp mattered to me. I cared much more about fitting in with the kids at home. Honestly, I enjoyed the positive attention I received at home on account of my disability. At camp, I was just another kid. Attending camp challenged my independence. I resented the constant supervision; if I could babysit my little sister, why couldn't I be left alone for five minutes? And I hated all of the rules. Lights had to be turned out at a certain time. Motorized wheelchairs had to be on low speed. Counselors had to hold on when we went down ramps and had to manually push us around the pool.

I'm not a bad kid. Why can't you just trust me?

My entire life was about fitting in and being a good kid, but I developed a bit of a rebellious attitude at camp. My behavior wasn't bad, but I constantly complained about the rules and activities. When at activities that didn't interest me, I read, which infuriated the counselors.

During the summer months when there was no camp, I was free of stupid rules and boring activities and actually enjoyed taking summer classes that helped me get ahead in school. One year I had a data entry job with the school district; this I enjoyed because the bosses treated me like an adult, not like a baby. And there was still time to go to the local swimming pool with Mom, where I could take a dip in the water or relax with a book. In the evening I went out for ice cream with friends and when I became interested in the opposite sex, cruised around the neighborhood in my chair "just happening" to pass by the homes of girls I liked.

As much as I disliked camp, my parents continued to send me for four more summers. Each year, I asked Mom if I had to go. "We'll see," she told me. But each summer, I wound up back at camp asking myself how I ended up in the same place. The year I had spinal fusion surgery, I convinced my parents that sleeping on a cot would be uncomfortable, which put an end to my annual misery.

There were off-season weekend retreats at camp, and though I balked at attending them because it just meant having to explain to yet another person how to best help me I did enjoy going. The retreats gave me a chance to see some of my friends with Duchenne in a more relaxed setting with informal activities like swimming. I looked forward to the opportunity to use the indoor pool because by then, the only way I could stand was in the water. Due to the fact that my legs were so contracted however, the water was up to my chin even in the shallow end of the pool. I was very unsteady on my feet but still enjoyed being in the water; that is until I nearly drowned.

Holding on to a rail to support myself in the pool, I was chatting with a friend when a clumsy mentally retarded camper bumped into me. I lost my balance and fell forward into the water, submerging my head. I tried to get up but couldn't; as my body bobbed up and down, I tried to lift my head above the water and catch my breath so I could tell my friend to call for help.

I can't get up! Oh no, please somebody help! I can't breathe!

But my friend already knew something was wrong and began screaming at the top of his lungs, "Counselor! Counselor! Help! Somebody help!" It seemed to take forever before someone heard him, and I began to wonder if anyone was ever going to get to me. Then just as I was about to lose consciousness, someone jumped in and grabbed me. The counselor quickly put me down on the pool deck where I caught my breath and began to cry. It was the scariest single moment of my life. My lungs were beginning to weaken, and had it been a couple of years later I may not have survived. That was the end of weekend retreats for me.

———— • ————

Fifth grade meant transitioning to another school. In our school district, four elementary schools fed into one middle school for grades five and six, which in turn fed into another middle school for seventh and eighth grades. Entering a new school meant new accessibility issues.

Several months earlier, I watched the school board on public access TV discuss whether a certain disabled student, me, might be better accommodated at a school for students with special needs. One board member expressed concern that because wheelchair access to one part of the building meant going outside and down a short path, my parents might sue if I got sick as a result of exposure to the cold weather. Though my parents assured me I would be able to go to the school, I was angry and a little scared that the board could make such arbitrary judgments.

You're not going to get out of this. I'm not leaving, so you're going to have to make things accessible!

As it turned out, we never had any problems with the school district and I began middle school that fall. A few weeks before school started, I again met with the school district's director of facilities and took a tour of the building to make sure the bathrooms, ramps, and special desks in each of my four classes met my needs.

One major accommodation, an elevator that would take me to the second floor wasn't ready the first year. While the elevator was under construction I monitored its progress, checking whenever possible with the school's maintenance director. In the absence of the elevator, all of my classes were assigned to first floor rooms. But even when the elevator was finally ready the next year, it sometimes malfunctioned. On one occasion it failed while I was on the second floor, and as a result four people carried me down two flights of stairs in my wheelchair. I was scared to death!

That was the year I began using adaptive technology on loan from the county's educational support unit. I received an Apple II GS and a color printer, as well as a primitive notebook-sized computer with a tiny LCD screen and a portable printer. Although I wasn't in desperate need of the equipment when I received it, the approval process was lengthy and there was uncertainty as to how long my dexterity would last. This way I had time to get used to the equipment before I would become completely dependent on it. I soon began using the computer to type my assignments, but was more impressed with being able to play games and print greeting cards, in color! My pediatrician, who owned an Apple, periodically came by to share software and helpful tips.

By virtue of the fact that middle school meant switching classes, I required assistance to open doors, retrieve books from my locker, and use the elevator. Thanks to her job in the school district, a friend's mom arranged for her son to assist me. We were assigned to just about every class together which was possible because we had similar academic abilities. Having one person help me was not necessarily the best idea because it became the basis of our friendship, and placed a great deal of pressure on him to be "responsible" for someone else. Regardless, we were practically inseparable and became best of friends.

Despite the new accommodations required, I continued to do well in school. I became aware of the world around me, avidly following current events; I knew of no other 11-year-old who subscribed to *Time!* Naturally, I was a whiz at my sixth grade teacher's weekly "Jeopardy" game. In English class, my ability to write was first recognized as I put my creative hat on each week and crafted a short story containing the week's spelling list.

While beginning to understand that there was little I could do to control the progression of my disease, one thing I did have control over was my effort in the classroom and I was downright arrogant about my ability to achieve in spite of my disease.

If I can do so well and I'm in a wheelchair, why can't other people?

A few years passed before I understood that I had a lot in my favor: a good family, an excellent education, and good medical care.

At least I had found a source of motivation. The more I achieved, the more it proved that someone with a disability could be as successful as someone without one. No matter what challenges I faced in the years to come, I would always take pride in my academic successes.

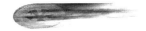

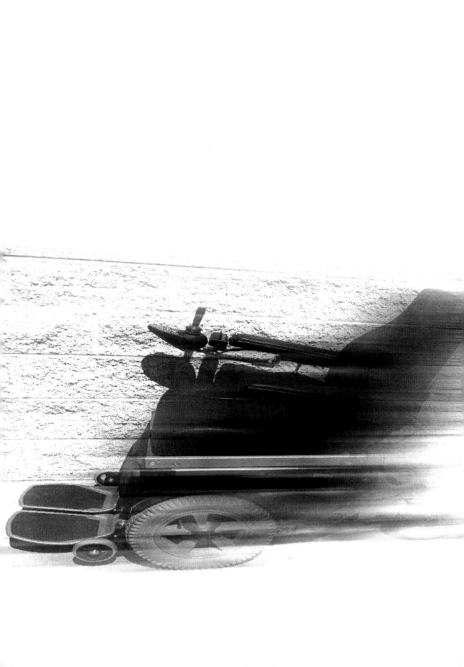

My Wonder Years

4

The screaming and yelling coming from the bathroom could be heard from across the house. It was shower night and Dad and I were arguing for a change.

I wanted things done a certain way and patience was not one of Dad's strong points. I complained about how he lifted me, the position of the shower chair, and the water temperature. He didn't like my tone of voice and told me so. I yelled at him; he yelled back.

After arguing back and forth several times I ended up back in my wheelchair smelling fresh as a daisy. I drove out of the bathroom shivering cold with tears streaming down my face, Dad wanting to tear the hair out of his head!

The more we fought the more Mom couldn't take it. Soon, she was giving me showers and taking care of just about all of my needs, including almost all of the lifting.

It was just easier for her to help me than to listen to Dad and me argue.

It upset me that Dad and I couldn't get along enough for him to help me, and that it led to a disproportionate burden on Mom. It was also normal. The fact that I had muscular dystrophy did not mean that everybody would somehow get along perfectly. Plus, I noticed that other boys with Duchenne also had one parent who was more involved helping them. In my case, it was Mom.

She and I typically saw eye-to-eye, so we had little reason to argue about how to do things. Mom was gentler and always took the extra step to make sure I was comfortable. When I was rude to her, she let me know.

"I don't have to do all this for you," she reminded me, "I can get Dad instead."

That shut me up real fast!

Having lost the ability to get out of my chair at all, I needed more help than before. I was no longer able to dress or bathe myself, and needed to be lifted in and out of bed, on and off the toilet. And most humiliating, I could no longer wipe myself.

Almost a teenager and I needed my mom to wipe my ass. I was too embarrassed to admit to even my family that I needed help with something so intimate. Eventually I accepted this newest loss of ability, and somehow blocked it out of my mind as it became routine.

My relationship with Dad had plenty of good moments despite our bathroom crises. The summer before I entered sixth grade, he picked me up from camp and couldn't wait to tell me that he and Mom had recently purchased a summer home in Brigantine, New Jersey, just north of Atlantic City. At night, I was able to look out my bedroom window and see the casino lights. Our house was a new one-story structure a block and a half from the beach. I wasn't able to go in the ocean and didn't enjoy baking in the hot sun, but none of that mattered. I loved when everyone went to the beach, leaving the place to me; I could kick back and play video games in air conditioned comfort. Mom always left me a snack, my urinal (not in the same place) and the telephone in case of emergency.

"Don't rush back," I told them.

Evenings were spent meandering across the island, gawking at million dollar homes and getting dessert at the local ice cream shop. I looked forward to getting up early in the morning and riding in my chair, with my sister Amy holding on to the handlebars. Burger King was our breakfast stop.

I enjoyed entertaining visiting guests, whether relatives or friends of the family, probably because we ate particularly well! Every time someone came to visit we enjoyed a veritable food fest. Weekends and holidays during the off-season were spent "down the shore" as well. The thought of spending time as a family was less than thrilling at the time, but our frequent trips offered a unique bonding opportunity.

Not that we didn't want to kill each other at times. While babysitting Stephanie, Amy and I often ended up screaming at one another. Once I even clipped her with my wheelchair out of frustration. She knew I didn't mean it, but I felt terrible and shocked at what I was capable of doing to someone with my wheelchair.

The lack of accessibility in the house eventually became an issue, as I had to take the leg rests off of my wheelchair to navigate the narrow hallway and couldn't get into the bathroom. After a few years, my parents sold our shore home. By then I was busy academically as a high school student; my sister's social life was full as well, making it more difficult to get away.

Thanks to the Starlight Foundation, an organization that granted wishes of sick and terminally ill children, we got away one February week. I was in sixth grade then, and the trip was to southern California where we had the opportunity to watch the filming of *The Wonder Years*," a weekly television family drama sitcom. The series was about a young boy, played by Fred Savage, growing up in the turbulent 1960s. After the filming, we met the cast of the show and were invited to join them for lunch on the set. They couldn't have been any friendlier, going out of their way to make us comfortable. It was surprising how down-to-earth everyone was compared to what one would have expected from Hollywood stars.

When first told about the trip I felt guilty, thinking that by my going someone very ill would miss out. I never considered myself sick; dying was not even on my radar screen.

I'm not really sick; I'm not dying. Do I really deserve this?

But who knew what kind of opportunities I would have in my life? There really was no telling how long I would live, and this was an opportunity to do something special while I still could.

In addition to visiting *The Wonder Years* set, we visited Universal Studios Hollywood theme park where I was fascinated by the parting of the Red Sea. We also toured the Los Angeles area, with stops on Rodeo Drive in Beverly Hills and in Malibu where we dined at a restaurant with a view of the Pacific Ocean. We also took a side trip south to San Diego and visited their nationally acclaimed zoo.

Smog and heavy traffic were not the only southern California phenomena we experienced. Sitting in our hotel room one evening, I felt a faint rumbling. I turned my head and saw something rather comical.

"Dad, why are you sliding toward the door?" I asked. At that moment we both realized what it was: an earthquake! The chandeliers were shaking and a housekeeper was crossing herself. Then just as quickly as it started, it was over. We flipped on the news and learned that there had indeed been an earthquake. This was one experience in California we all could have lived without.

I was grateful for the opportunity to visit California and thoroughly enjoyed the trip, but now it was time to get back to my life. Upon returning home, the attention I received at school was a little embarrassing. One Fred Savage-crazed girl in my English class was especially excited.

That fall, I entered seventh grade. Even though it meant moving to another school, there were few accessibility issues to work out. Built in the early 1970s, the school was the district's newest building; it already had an elevator and just about every entrance was level, eliminating the need for ramps. I no longer had just one student helping me. Although there was no set schedule, I could count on friends in just about every class to hand me a book from my bag, escort me on the elevator, and assist me in the bathroom. I realized however that it was becoming more difficult to count on friends, as they had other friends and things they wanted to do during recess besides staying inside with me. Sometimes, I had to resort to "guilting" people into assisting me.

"Would you mind helping me during lunch period? There's no one else I can ask," I would say.

I was pretty good at it and had no real alternative, but it felt wrong. I wished there was a staff member to assist me on a regular basis. That way, my friends could be friends rather than helpers.

The transition to a new school had no effect on my schoolwork, especially judging from the number of phone calls I received from classmates seeking homework help. I beamed with pride, knowing that my peers respected me for my intelligence. I was no longer just "the kid in the wheelchair."

Apparently the only person who was not impressed was my art teacher who unceremoniously awarded me with a 'C' one period, ruining my otherwise straight-A report card. When Mom called to protest, the old curmudgeon told her that my work was only "average."

It's just art appreciation class, you asshole! You show up and try your best, and you get an A.

With success came the pressure to keep it up. By now my expectations pushed me far more than my parents. I enjoyed the satisfaction of getting good grades, although there were times the pressure got to me.

It was no wonder I constantly suffered from migraine headaches. I often came home from school and went straight to bed. The blinds had to be drawn, the lights turned out and my bedroom door closed. The slightest sounds bothered me. Eventually I threw up, which temporarily helped, but did little to relieve the intense pounding in my right temple. On one day following such a headache, I had the added stress of making up the homework I had been unable to complete the night before.

I also suffered from a nervous stomach. At one school dance, I had a sudden case of the runs. Completely embarrassed, I had no choice but to ask the vice principal to lift me onto the toilet. It was a memory I hoped to forget!

Academic pressure was not the sole cause of my stress. Entering my teens made it increasingly important to fit in. I constantly worried about what others thought and felt the need to prove that despite my wheelchair I was just like everyone else.

Getting noticed by girls was a major source of frustration. I felt the main reason for this particular problem was the fact that I was in a wheelchair. Girls seemed to think that I was just a nice guy, and didn't see me in any other light. I was devastated one Valentine's Day when I didn't receive a single "candy-gram."

Am I that big of a loser? Honestly, I don't know why I even bother to go to school with normal people.

Of course, I never put myself out there either and was much too shy to send out Valentine messages of my own. I liked myself, but was sure that none of the girls I liked would be interested in a guy in a wheelchair. The one time a girl did have a crush on me I largely ignored her, although I was actually flattered. She was a relative of a family friend and a fellow writer on the school paper, but I was too interested in other girls who were not interested in me.

As much as I wanted to be noticed by the opposite sex, the last thing I wanted was to stick out like a sore thumb on account of my disability. Sitting in social studies class one afternoon I tried to get closer to my desk when my foot got stuck between my desk and the front tire of my wheelchair, twisting my knee. I screamed out in pain, interrupting the class and scaring the teacher half to death. I was taken to the nurse's office, Mom came to pick me up, and the next few days were spent in agony. I was much more upset about the spectacle I had created in front of everybody.

Yeah, crying is real mature. Now everyone thinks I'm a big baby.

I found this ironic in that I was about to become a man

according to the Jewish faith at the traditional Bar Mitzvah ceremony.

After spending nearly a year preparing, the big day finally arrived. In a chapel packed with family and friends, I chanted a part of the Torah that I had learned and practiced repeatedly. Though I sung in school choirs I was nervous about singing solo, especially in front of my friends. But I threw caution to the wind and went ahead anyway, telling myself that some of my friends had much worse voices!

For my parents, grandparents, aunts and uncles, the occasion was symbolic of the fact that I had reached this point in spite of the challenges in my life. In a speech Dad gave at the end of the ceremony, he told me I had demonstrated that someone in a wheelchair could be as "bright, creative and productive as anyone else."

Then it was time to celebrate. My parents held a lavish affair in my honor at a nearby country club, complete with a band and a caricaturist to draw portraits of my friends. More than 150 guests attended, including about 30 of my friends from school and synagogue. The festive night was filled with food, music, dancing, and games like "The Limbo" and "Coke and Pepsi" for the kids. I relished being the man of the hour, enjoying the female attention, hugs and kisses I received. Then just like that, the best day of my young life was over.

For the remainder of the school year and part of the next year my life was dominated by the Bar Mitzvah "circuit," with an event nearly every Saturday. I visited several synagogues and almost every country club in the area, which led to the inevitable accessibility questions. Mom made sure I could get into the various facilities. If bus transportation was provided to shuttle kids from the synagogue to the country club, Dad picked me up in our van.

It was one of the rare times I actually had a social life. I enjoyed the opportunity to interact with my friends outside of school. At times I even got out on the dance floor, though driving my wheelchair in coordination with everyone else during the "Electric Slide" was a bit of a challenge. The trick was not killing anyone in the process!

But just like at school, it was difficult to be noticed by girls. I watched them fawn over certain guys, dance with them, and touch them. I was so jealous.

What's so great about them? I'm good-looking and probably smarter, too.

I didn't see myself defined by my wheelchair, so I couldn't understand why girls weren't interested in me.

The one time I did receive the attention I craved, I ended up with a broken leg! It happened at the Bat Mitzvah of a girl I had known since preschool.

"Come on, dance with me," she said. My face turned beet red.

She's the Bat Mitzvah girl. How can I say no?

"Uh...well...uh...sure," I stammered.

"Can I sit on your lap?" she asked when we got out on the dance floor. Something told me it wasn't a good idea, but how could I say no?

"Uh...yeah...well, I guess."

I should have trusted my instinct. With the leg rests on my wheelchair, my legs were elevated from the seat cushion with no support underneath. I didn't have much muscle strength left, so the bone was left to support her weight even though it was not much. After a few seconds I felt an intense throbbing pain in my right thigh, but said nothing. After she got off my lap, the pain actually grew worse. When my parents and sisters came to pick me up for a weekend trip to the shore, I approached the van with tears streaming down my face.

"What's wrong?" Mom asked with concern.

"My leg, my leg, I think I hurt my leg," I sobbed. It really hurt, but none of us believed anything was seriously wrong. I had hurt myself before and made a big deal about it, only to feel better a few days later. We tried applying ice to my leg and wrapping it, which did provide some relief. But the pain was excruciating when Dad picked me up to put me in bed. It was a miserable weekend for everyone.

Upon returning home, we went to a local hospital for x-rays. The results indicated a fracture. Since I was already being followed by an orthopedist at CHOP, we went to the muscular dystrophy clinic there the next day. My leg hurt so badly that I was scared to death to let anyone touch it. After the x-rays confirmed a fracture, I received a blue (my choice) fiberglass cast that ran from the top of my thigh down to my toes.

A broken bone was not the end of the world, but it was upsetting. I took care of my body with pride despite my disease, and worried that my leg might not heal and look the same. But the clinic nurse reassured me that some of the boys I knew with Duchenne had broken bones before and had healed perfectly.

The entire incident was almost as bad for the girl who had sat on my lap. Not only did she feel guilty about hurting me, she had to put up with all of the gossip and jokes. I didn't blame her, nor was I angry at her. After all, it was my choice to dance with her. Plus, no other girl had ever asked me to dance before, which I did not forget.

Now, I was more concerned with getting better. The cast on my leg made me heavier and more awkward to lift. I was also growing, so lifting me was starting to strain Mom's back. Even before I broke my leg a physical therapist had recommended obtaining a Hoyer lift, which was essentially a crane attached to a u-shaped base that opened to fit around a wheelchair. I would sit on a nylon "sling" attached to the lift with chains. When it was delivered, Mom and I took one look at the contraption and stuck it in a corner.

Pain or no pain, it just seemed easier to lift me. Eventually, we reconsidered. Usually resistant to change, I was not against it. I was not even afraid of hanging in the air. As it turned out, we both really liked using the lift. After a couple of weeks, Mom was an old pro. It didn't really take any more time in my routine, and because the sling had a cut-out I could hover over the toilet to do my business.

We later obtained a bathtub clamp so the lift could be

used to hold me while I showered. After showering I needed to get back into my wheelchair, freezing cold on the wet sling, and then into bed so the sling could be removed.

It was around this time that I also got a hospital bed. I was completely embarrassed.

I'm not a sick person. I don't need this. I don't want it.

Still, I had to admit that it was kind of cool to move my head and feet up and down whenever I felt like it. I just wasn't about to brag about it to my friends.

From a medical standpoint, I was doing well. I had good use of my hands with enough dexterity to use a needle and thread in home economics class, and could still raise my arms above my head. However, my doctors were concerned about my weight. In less than a year, I had gained 19 pounds. Too much weight would put added stress on my heart and lungs.

I'm not fat. I'm not going on a diet. I already can't walk; now I can't eat like everyone else?

My parents agreed to keep an eye on things, but I was glad that they didn't make me change my eating habits. It was probably just a growth spurt anyway because from that point forward my weight remained stable.

I began seeing a pulmonologist at the hospital when I was 12, and other than my weight increase he was pleased with my condition. I was rarely short of breath, though I sometimes felt unusually tired. Occasionally, I had trouble swallowing food. Over the next few years, my pulmonary function tests, which measured the strength and capacity of my lungs, indicated that while I was growing predictably weaker, my respiratory status was good for someone my age with Duchenne.

The doctor did have me begin using an inspirometer, a small plastic device with a narrow, clear chamber connected to a short tube with a mouthpiece at the end. When I inhaled, a yellow cup rose inside the chamber. The goal was to keep the cup up as long as possible. At times I was very vigilant about using the "breathing thing," as I called it, but at other times I neglected it for weeks on end.

Around this time, my pediatrician began prescribing antibiotics whenever I caught a cold to ensure that I didn't develop pneumonia. While antibiotics would not cure the common cold, they could prevent a secondary infection that might lead to pneumonia.

The only other concern was scoliosis, or curvature of my spine. Should it worsen, it would adversely affect me from a respiratory standpoint. This was not an issue that needed to be addressed just yet, but it wasn't long thereafter that it would need attention.

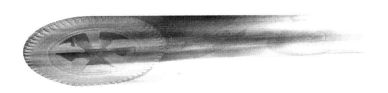

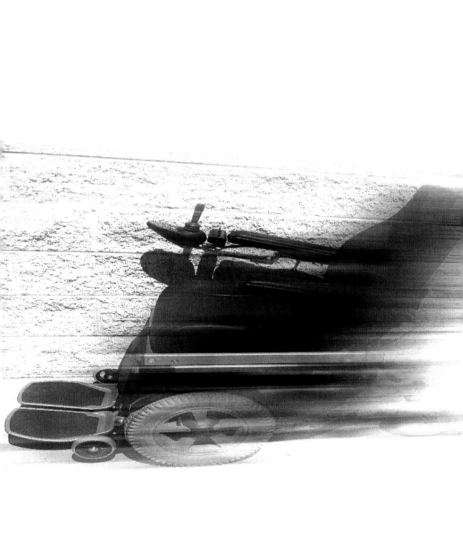

No Pain, No Gain

5

After spending all morning at the muscular dystrophy clinic for a checkup, my parents and I were getting hungry and cranky. All we had to do was see the orthopedist and we could get out of there and back to our routine.

Earlier I had undergone routine x-rays to track the progression of my scoliosis. I knew that some of the other guys with Duchenne had undergone spinal fusion surgery to correct the problem. Hopefully it was something I wouldn't need because it sounded painful! Why would I? Aside from some occasional lower back pain, I felt fine and was convinced that I was doing better than the other guys I knew.

As we sat in the examining room, five minutes passed then 10, 15, and 30. What was keeping the doctor so long? We all had better things to do than sit around all day.

If we get out of here soon, I can still get to school for a few classes. I can eat lunch on the way.

As Dad spotted the doctor coming down the hallway, we collectively sighed. Surely we would be out of there in no time at all. But that all changed the second the doctor strolled into the room.

"It's time," he said in a booming Charlton Heston-like voice. With that, Mom and I both burst into tears. We knew what the doctor meant; my scoliosis had reached the point where I needed surgery.

But it wasn't only curvature of my spine that determined surgery was necessary now, according to the doctor. If my respiratory status declined much further, which was inevitable in my disease, the lengthy surgery would be too risky.

The operation would help prevent serious problems. If the scoliosis continued unchecked, my body would likely twist into an abnormal position, making it difficult to sit comfortably in my wheelchair. The back pain I was experiencing would worsen, and of greater concern it would be more difficult to expand my lungs, making me more susceptible to developing pneumonia. At this point, I had not yet suffered any serious respiratory illnesses, but would have a better chance of avoiding them if I had the operation now.

Even at 14 years old when it was hard to think about the future, I perfectly understood the justification for the surgery. It still didn't make the prospect of having it any easier. Maybe surgery was an everyday occurrence for the doctor, but it was a big deal for me and for my parents.

It was difficult to believe I needed something so drastic when I basically felt fine. My disease had always been serious, but this was the first time in my life that it required an invasive treatment.

As we left the hospital that day, the muscular dystrophy clinic nurse we had known since my earliest days as a patient there tried to offer some words of encouragement.

"You'll sit straighter, your clothes will fit better, and you won't get sick," she told me.

Maybe it won't be so bad after all. She's seen the other kids who have had the surgery, so she must know what she's talking about!

The effect of her encouragement only lasted a short time. As the mid-February surgery date approached, my apprehension grew.

"I'm nervous," I told Mom at least once a day, not exactly sure what I was apprehensive about other than the unknown. Though I had undergone the muscle biopsy ten years earlier, I didn't really know what it was like to have surgery or to stay in the hospital. Moreover, it was the thought of how much pain the surgery would cause that worried me the most.

A few weeks prior to the surgery I spent an afternoon at the hospital, traveling throughout the building for standard preoperative tests like x-rays and an echocardiogram. Blood was taken and stored because I was likely to lose much of it during surgery. We later asked family members with my blood type to donate additional blood. Although the supply was considered HIV-safe there was no guarantee and we didn't want to take any chances, slim as they might have been.

I've already got muscular dystrophy. I don't need AIDS, too!

My parents met with the surgeon to learn more about the operation. A long incision would be made down the center of my back, from the bottom of my neck to my tailbone. Holes would be drilled in my pelvis for placement of metal rods. These rods would then be connected to the vertebrae on both sides of my spine using wires and be tensioned properly, which would correct the scoliosis. The bone fragments removed to make way for the wires would be grafted between the vertebrae, so that over time the vertebrae would fuse together making my spine more stable. I would actually "grow" an inch or so taller as a result of the surgery. However, I would be less flexible, unable to bend from the middle of my back.

Although I wanted time to go slowly, inevitably it did not. As my classmates enjoyed ski trips over Presidents' Weekend, I checked into the hospital for surgery. The night before the surgery, a doctor came into my room to discuss a few issues. First, he explained that to help me breathe during surgery a tube would be inserted down my throat. He wanted me to be prepared for the possibility that the tube would still be in my throat when I woke up. If that was the case I would be unable to speak, but this was no need to panic.

The doctor also explained that to control my pain afterwards I would be given a PCA, or patient-controlled-administration device. Within a prescribed limit, I could push a button placed in my hand to administer myself more pain medication. With barely enough strength left in my fingers, I hoped I would be able to push the button.

Finally, the choice was mine as to the method used to administer the anesthetic that would be used to put me asleep. It could be given intravenously or inhaled through a mask placed over my nose and mouth. Although I hardly enjoyed needles, I quickly opted for the IV method. The thought of having a mask held over my face scared me, as I imagined the feeling of suffocation.

Early the next morning I was wheeled into pre-op slightly drowsy from the light sedative I had been given, nervous but fascinated by the whole process of having surgery. Various doctors and nurses spoke with me and my parents. To monitor spinal cord function, electrodes were glued to my head. I was told that someone would be paying close attention to this aspect of my condition throughout the procedure.

Saying little to my parents before being wheeled off to surgery, I knew these final moments were probably more difficult for them than for me. I was apprehensive, but only in the sense that the hospital personnel around me seemed to indicate how serious the situation was. Even as a child I was aware of the risks of the surgery but still couldn't imagine not waking afterwards.

When I was finally wheeled into the operating room,

an IV was inserted in the back of one of my hands. It didn't hurt much because I was too busy asking that they warn me right before administering anesthesia so I could count how long it took to fall asleep.

The next thing I remembered was waking up after surgery.

Damn it, they didn't let me count!

Then I realized how stupid I was.

I was worried about this for so long. It's over... I really did it!

I noticed that it was totally dark in the room or so it seemed that way, and wondered where everyone was. It was so quiet.

"Hello," I called out as best I could.

Eventually, a nurse came over. I didn't know exactly what to say. Here was a woman who had obviously been monitoring me, but we had never met.

"Where are my parents?" I asked.

"They went home for the night," she explained.

Oh... Wow. I must have been asleep the entire day! That's so weird — I've lost a whole day of my life.

She told me to go back to sleep, and that was enough for me. When I woke up again it was morning and my parents were there, and so was the pain, an intense throbbing that radiated up and down my back. My chest was also sore, especially around my rib cage, the result of how I had been positioned on the operating table. I stayed awake for a few minutes before falling back to sleep. It was the first time in my life that I remembered not feeling fully alert, and learned just how much I disliked the feeling of not being in control. For much of my life, I had not had complete control of my body, so it was important for me to have complete control over my mental faculties. Now that I was not fully alert, I felt completely helpless.

The first few days in intensive care were most difficult in that sense. I completely lost track of time, and just wanted to sleep so the pain would go away. But it seemed that no one wanted to leave me alone. Just as I became comfortable, an x-ray technician came and slid a hard metal plate under my throbbing back. Doctors touched my extremities to make sure I still had feeling in them. Nurses collected blood samples. Physical therapists wanted to move my arms and legs. All were necessary interruptions but they seemed endless, and the last thing I wanted was to be touched.

Just leave me alone. I'm in so much pain.

For much of my stay in the hospital, I was unable to urinate or move my bowels, a nasty little side effect of anesthesia. The tremendous discomfort I experienced in my abdomen as a result just added to the excruciating pain in my back and the soreness in my chest. It was at this point that I received my indoctrination to the wonderful world of catheters and laxatives. Though I was assured by nurse and doctor alike that my normal bowel and bladder function would soon resume, it was hard to believe them. For a while, it seemed that I would never be able to go to the bathroom on my own again. Forget the embarrassment; the solutions to these problems were downright unpleasant.

There's no way that anyone is jamming a tube into my penis for the rest of my life. That part of my anatomy is not designed to work that way!

The tremendous pain in my back was worse than anything and I was in total agony after one sleepless night of pain. I hit the button on the PCA over and over again without obtaining any noticeable relief. It was impossible to push the nurse call button because my right hand had the PCA in it, and I didn't have enough strength in my left hand to hold anything. The door to my room was closed to help me sleep, so calling out for help was not an option. It seemed like I had been in pain for hours on end, and could do nothing but stare at the wall and moan as the throbbing in my back intensified. When Mom arrived some time later, she found me hysterically sobbing. I'm not sure what was eventually administered to bring my pain under control, but knew that I never wanted to experience pain like that again.

Though I understood the importance of the surgery, I found few positives about the overall hospital experience. The nurses were friendly but not especially helpful. My parents had to get me in and out of bed. When the nurses were caring for me, I was afraid they might abruptly move my legs which I could no longer straighten. I was not the least bit interested in letting them bathe me; cleanliness was hardly a pressing issue to me the way I felt.

As skilled as they were, the doctors seemed highly insensitive. When the surgeon and his underlings visited to check my progress, my parents and I were all but ignored. They seemed unconcerned about my overall condition, especially the pain I was experiencing. As long as the surgery was successful, everything else seemed a minor issue for them. Worse yet, some were even ignorant of my disease.

A few days after surgery, a young doctor cleared me to get out of bed. "Go ahead. Hop on up," he told me. My parents were incredulous. Mom explained, "Well, he can't do that by himself. It's going to take us a few minutes."

I was not angry. I just couldn't believe doctors could be so clueless and insensitive.

A week after the surgery, I was released from the hospital. As much as I hated being in the hospital, I did not want to leave.

How could I possibly be ready to go? Is it really safe for me to leave? What about the pain?

Mom helped me get dressed and then left me with Dad, who had driven separately in our van. Waiting as he put down the wheelchair lift, I was freezing in the 30-degree weather. Despite being unable to twist my body to look behind me, I managed to back onto the lift. When it reached the van floor, I began to slowly back up.

A loud "clunk" could be heard, as a throbbing pain went down the back of my head.

What the hell...oh, the extra inch. I must be too tall!

The van had a raised roof, but not a raised doorway.

"Dad!"

"What?!"

"I can't get in! What are we going to do?"

Do something. Hurry up already! I'm so cold.

He thought for a moment and then tipped my wheelchair backwards and manually wheeled me into the van. It worked but I dreaded the thought of getting out when we got home.

Riding in the van was awkward. My body was so rigid that there was no give when we hit bumps on the road. It was more uncomfortable at high speeds, but as Dad pointed out we were on the expressway. "What would you like me to do?" he asked.

I wanted to get home fast regardless of the bumps and pain. I held my breath for practically the entire trip, terrified of damaging my back, as unlikely a possibility as that may have been. It was hard to feel confident that something so new was safe to be bounced around in a vehicle.

The first couple weeks at home were absolutely awful. I was still in a considerable amount of pain and had trouble sleeping comfortably. It seemed that every other minute, I needed help with something. I was irritable and impatient. Sitting in my wheelchair was impossible for longer than twenty minutes at a time, and as a result I needed to be transferred from my bed to my wheelchair and back several times a day.

This put a tremendous strain on Mom, not only physically but emotionally as well. I was not an only child and my sisters also required her attention. Dad had to resume working but when he was at home, Mom grew angry with him for not doing enough for me. When he tried to help me, I was highly resistant to his efforts. Unfortunate for both of us, he was unfamiliar with my needs and I was too tired to explain. Furthermore, Dad had never reacted well to taking direction from me.

Five days after I was discharged from the hospital, it was Mom's birthday. The following week, I turned 15. Safe to say, neither one of us felt much like celebrating. Even for a stable family like ours, the initial stages of my recovery at home proved to be more stressful than any of us had ever anticipated.

As successful as the surgery eventually proved, I doubted the doctors could ever have fully appreciated the immediate impact it had on members of my family. I vowed to never have surgery or go in the hospital again. I simply didn't want to experience the physical or emotional pain, and had become skeptical of the practicality of treatments prescribed by doctors.

One thing that did help me get through this time was baseball. In need of a distraction from pain, I began watching the Philadelphia Phillies' spring training games. The team that had not experienced a winning season in several years actually began to win games.

As the team's fortunes improved, so did mine. I was gradually able to sit in my wheelchair for longer periods of time. It turned out that my first year following the team would be one of the most memorable seasons in team history, though it ended with a heartbreaking loss in the World Series that fall.

The attention I received from friends and family also helped during my recovery. For a while, people came every day, many bearing food and other get-well gifts.

Sometimes visitors arrived when they were least expected. One afternoon, the doorbell rang as Mom was wheeling me out of the bathroom on the Hoyer lift. Naked from the waist down, I nearly had a heart attack when she looked out the window and told me it was a girl I had a serious crush on.

"Quick! Put me in my chair!" I yelled.

Once I was in my wheelchair, she headed for the door. "No, no, no...Wait! Cover me up first!" I shouted.

Throughout the entire ordeal of major surgery, I was never as scared as I was at that moment. Nothing could have been worse than being embarrassed in front of a girl I liked. I was no different from any other teenager in that regard.

Not that being half-dressed was the worst thing either. While recovering I would often put a blanket over my legs rather than wearing pants, which drew some good-natured ribbing from a mixed group of friends who came to visit me. "What's with the blanket?" one of them said with a smirk.

"Wouldn't you like to know?" I teased.

It was nice to have a moment of levity because having surgery was an endless ordeal. Seemingly minor details like having the stitches removed from my back proved extremely painful. "This isn't going to hurt a lot, is it?" I asked the doctor, dreading the answer.

"It shouldn't be too bad," he said nonchalantly.

With that, he proceeded to rip the stitches right out of my back as I screamed in pain and my eyes watered.

Not hurt that bad? On what planet? You obviously must have a different interpretation of pain than I do.

Follow-up x-rays were equally painful, as I had to be lifted out of my wheelchair. At home, I tolerated using the Hoyer lift without much pain because it sat me up gradually and then held me in a steady position. But it wasn't possible to use it for x-rays as the base of the lift did not fit under the table, so Dad picked me up instead.

Whenever lifted, I was at the mercy of the person lifting me. My comfort could not be ensured, as the person had to be more focused on not dropping me. Normally, it wouldn't have been such a problem, but the area between my lower back and upper thighs was extremely tight, which I assumed was because the rod in my back had been screwed into my pelvis. When my thighs were elevated, I felt intense pain in my lower back.

Aside from the pain endured in the weeks and months after surgery, many small physical tasks had to be learned again. Prior to surgery, I had leaned against the table to feed myself because I no longer had the strength to lift my arm to raise a fork or spoon to my mouth. Now that I could no longer bend from the middle of my back, I was concerned about being able to feed myself again. As a 15-

year-old trying not to draw any additional attention to myself especially at school, needing someone to feed me would be devastating. The last thing I wanted was to look like a helpless baby. It was just a few years earlier that I was the one feeding my baby sister.

Using as many as three telephone books I figured out how to position myself in such a way that I could still reach my mouth with a fork; using a knife was no longer possible. Over time, I learned to do without any phone books, found new ways to type at the computer, turn the pages of books, write with a pen, and perform many other tasks I had taken for granted.

My inability to bend from the middle of my back also required that I learn a different way to enter our van. The medical equipment company was able to lower my wheelchair seat slightly, but that didn't completely solve the problem. Eventually, I taught myself to cock my head to the right, just enough to clear the doorway. It took some practice as my first instinct was to bend from the middle of my back, which didn't work and caused a great deal of discomfort.

After being home for a couple weeks, it was time to start catching up on schoolwork. I had anticipated the school district hiring tutors to help me, but to my surprise most of my major subject teachers agreed to tutor me at home. I was grateful for their kindness, as it certainly was not required by the school. As a result, from an academic standpoint I was up to speed.

As winter gave way to spring I continued to build up

my energy level slowly but surely, and by mid-April was well enough to return to school. Teachers, classmates and friends welcomed me back. The same girl who had unexpectedly visited me at home was so excited to see me that she gave me a great big bear-hug, which scared me since I didn't know if it could hurt my back. I blushed out of embarrassment, but was thrilled as it was one of the rare instances that a girl had ever touched me!

Even though the tutoring I had received at home had indeed kept me up to date with my studies, I found it difficult to maintain my energy level. At first, I attended school for only half days and on some days came home to lie in bed for an hour.

Will I ever regain the energy I used to have?

Little by little my old self returned and I was pretty much back to normal by the end of the school year. It amazed me how the body could heal from such trauma, especially *my* body, which was not healthy in the first place.

My health remained stable for the next several years with the exception of semi-occasional bouts with constipation. Even though my disease primarily affected cardiac and skeletal muscles, the muscles in the gastrointestinal tract were also affected. For me, there could not have been a more embarrassing aspect of my disease. At times, I was in such discomfort that I was unable to concentrate on school work. I even stayed home from school sometimes, as laughable as it seemed. Tired and irritable, the last thing I wanted to think about was interacting with other people.

My entire personality revolved around being upbeat and hiding any problems I had, but it was tough being myself when I was so uncomfortable. Upon returning to school I never let Mom reveal the true reason for my absence in excuse notes, making sure that she attributed it to a much less embarrassing "upset stomach" instead.

All I could picture was being a substitute actor in the laxative commercial for the middle-aged man whose wife embarrassed him by loudly discussing his problem in public.

"...You know, the other day when you missed school because you were CONSTIPATED?!"

Not that there wasn't anything funny about my problem. One particular occurrence resolved itself on the same night I watched the Phillies clinch the National League pennant in nail-biting fashion. I guess I clinched as well! I was not sure which event was more satisfying.

I was fortunate that constipation was my worst problem, as opposed to something more serious like pneumonia which is always a risk for someone with Duchenne. Though uncomfortable, it was merely an inconvenience. Still, if I had been less embarrassed about it, I would have been more proactive when this seemingly innocuous problem threatened my life several years later.

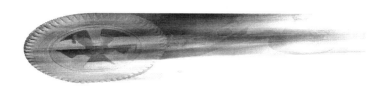

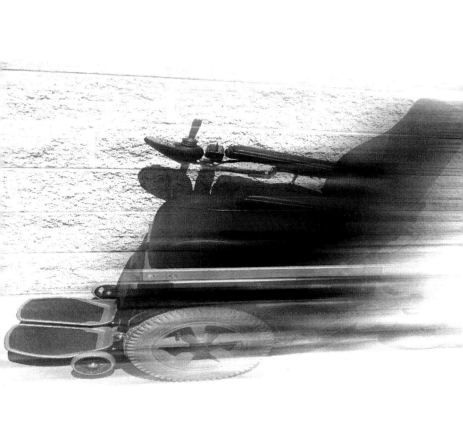

Just Like Everyone Else

6

As I sat in the cool dark auditorium, listening to faculty and administrators welcome the class of 1996 to Cheltenham High School, I found it hard to fathom that graduation and the real world were less than four years away.

It was exciting to look ahead, but a little scary as well. I assumed that when the time came, I would go to college like everyone else. Still, I couldn't help wondering how my health would be by then. It was hard to imagine being any different from the way I was now, although a lot could change in four years.

But then I was getting ahead of myself. All I really needed to worry about right now was getting used to high school.

As usual when I entered another school in the district, accommodations were required to make the building accessible. The only significant expense for the school district was the installation of an elevator. Neither one of the two most commonly used entrances was wheelchair accessible, but I was able to enter the building through a rarely used entrance.

Once inside, I had to drive my wheelchair up a steep ramp that was originally designed for moving equipment to the nearby auditorium. It seemed strange entering the building like a piece of cargo, but I really didn't mind. Getting inside was the key, and that was good enough for me.

Because the stalls in the restrooms were too small for me to fit inside, I was permitted to use the bathroom inside the coaches' locker room. Unfortunately, it was located at the farthest corner of the school. If I was on the first floor, I needed to take the elevator; and if on the second floor, it still took some time to get there. In most cases I was able to time things just right, leaving one class a few minutes early, stopping at the bathroom and arriving a few minutes late to my next class.

One drawback was that at times I would be in midstream when the door to the locker room suddenly flung open and one of the coaches entered. This would cause me to tense up, unable to finish peeing.

"Hey, Josh! How ya doin'?" the offending coach would greet me.

How does it look like I'm doing? I'm trying to take a piss here. Do you mind?

In the classroom, I required few accommodations. Only able to elevate my arm slightly and extend the pen in my hand, I needed teachers to make sure that they glanced in my direction during class discussions. I always sat in the front row but it still took some effort for teachers to remember to look my way.

I was able to take notes and tests without assistance, and though I wrote more slowly than my classmates, completing quizzes and tests in the time allotted was never a problem. Had I been given extra time, other students might have complained that I had an unfair advantage. Still, being permitted to use a tape recorder in case I grew tired of writing was great.

For the first time the school district assigned an aide to provide assistance during the course of the school day. I was thrilled, having grown tired of depending on friends and classmates for help in previous years. Now I didn't have to worry about who would help me get books out of my locker, put on my coat, or hand me my urinal in the bathroom. The aide also had to help unzip my pants, as well as empty and clean my urinal. I definitely would have felt uncomfortable asking my friends to help me with such tasks. Depending on the class, I either had the aide sit with me, or more typically help me get my books out for class before leaving me on my own.

Having someone paid to assist me was a learning experience, particularly from a personality standpoint. During my sophomore and junior years, an often cantankerous, semi-retired man served as my aide. Although anyone who interacted with him was subjected to a constant stream of complaints, I had to deal with his moodiness on a daily basis. Taking the high road, I did my best to be pleasant and appreciative of his assistance even though it was frustrating.

Why is it okay for him to be miserable but not me? Who's the adult here?

Of course, there was little to be gained by responding to his attitude; in the eyes of faculty members this would have been seen as disrespectful and might have led to my aide becoming even more unpleasant and uncooperative. At times, I did make snide comments under my breath. Some of my teachers sensed my frustration and allowed me to vent my feelings to them.

As annoying as this was at times, I never insisted on a replacement. I figured he wasn't really doing anything horrible and that asking for someone to replace him would be more trouble than it was worth.

Thankfully Mom did not feel the same way and insisted that the school district find someone different to help me during my senior year. As a result, they hired an extremely affable, grandfatherly man who was retired from the Air Force. Talking with him about all the places in the world he had traveled during his career was fascinating.

With the necessary accommodations in place I was able to concentrate on my school work. I enjoyed the taste of success with each assignment, paper, or test. My motivation to succeed also came from attending school with so many intelligent classmates. The best way to earn their respect was to demonstrate that I could do just as well.

It was also important to prove to teachers that I wasn't

just someone who needed to be accommodated, but a dedicated student who wanted to be treated like everyone else. Each year I suspected that at least a few teachers wondered if I was looking for a break from them, but by the end of the school year I knew I had gained their respect. At the same time however, I still worried that other students would see me as a teacher's pet which certainly would not have won friends.

Although successful in the classroom, I continued to lack confidence in my academic abilities. There were better all-around students. I was much stronger in English and history than in science or math. Yet I always felt the need to prove that I belonged in honors classes despite my disability. This was not entirely bad, as I never took success for granted and worked hard, even though it probably made life more stressful than necessary.

Though earning good grades was an obsession, I genuinely enjoyed learning. I especially loved American history class. As a person with a disability, I identified with the ideals our country represented. If I worked hard enough, I had as good a chance to succeed as the next person despite my physical shortcomings. The fact that America often failed to live up to its high standards was tough to understand. I personally hadn't experienced any significant oppression in my life, but knew how frustrating and hurtful it could be when something was inaccessible.

Immigration, the Great Depression and subsequent New Deal, the Red Scare and the Civil Rights Movement greatly interested me. I came to believe that while people needed to be responsible, it was also necessary that government do its part to ensure that everyone had a chance to succeed.

Beyond the classroom, I made an effort to participate in some of the extracurricular activities offered at the school, with varying degrees of success. I wanted to do more with my life than obsess over assignments and books, and also wanted to show people that I was determined to take advantage of every opportunity available.

In two subsequent years I auditioned for the annual school play without success. Hardly the most skilled actor, I still found it hard to believe that my attempt at acting was so bad I couldn't have been cast in a minor role. Being rejected for talent was something I understood and accepted, but was convinced that I was not chosen because I was in a wheelchair.

The school's performing arts program was so professional that having someone in a wheelchair would have taken away from it. I certainly wouldn't have looked the part, whatever it might have been. Just getting me on stage would have been challenging from an accessibility standpoint. It was just easier to reject me. Had I questioned the decision, the teachers would have said that it was based on talent, and no one would have been able to challenge something so subjective. What frustrated me the most was that minds were made up before I even began to audition; I never even had a shot, regardless of how hard I tried.

I was able to get involved in student government, chosen to serve on the student council's executive committee, which planned school activities. I relished the opportunity to contribute to something that benefited the entire student body. It certainly felt much better than spending every moment thinking about myself.

In senior year, I considered running for president of the student council. Had I been elected, I would have had to attend all school activities and of course, someone would have to be there to assist with my bathroom needs. It also would have resulted in depending on my parents for transportation.

After talking myself out of the idea several times, I summoned the courage to attend an exploratory meeting. At the end of the meeting, the faculty advisor pulled me aside. "I'm not trying to discourage you, but are you sure you want to do this? You do realize the responsibilities?" he asked.

With that, the wind went out of my sails. His concerns were valid and were the very reason I had been talking myself out of running in the first place. Now I was being talked out of it by someone else. My ability to commit was being questioned on account of my disability.

Don't you think I realize what kind of commitment is involved? I would sooner die than let people down.

Maybe a job like that was a bit of a reach, but I vowed that I would never again allow myself to be talked out of anything I wanted to do.

I was able to demonstrate commitment through my

work for the school newspaper, *The Cheltonian*. As a freshman, I expressed an interest in writing for the paper despite the fact that the staff was mostly composed of seniors. I loved that it was a real, live newspaper. The tiny office where the paper was produced contained state-of-the-art equipment with computers, a laser printer, and a flatbed scanner.

Writing mostly news and feature articles, I took great pride in asking good questions and crafting informative, organized, mistake-free articles that were submitted on time. I felt if I was unreliable, fellow staff members would think that someone in a wheelchair could not be trusted.

I enjoyed my work on the newspaper so much that by sophomore year, I decided to pursue a career in journalism. Yet I did not have a whole lot of confidence in my writing ability and often deferred to other staff members. This was the main reason I never sought to be an editor, in addition to the fact that such a position would have meant longer hours and require more flexibility in my schedule in terms of transportation, eating, and using the bathroom.

I had my chance to be a leader outside of school when I was elected president of my synagogue's confirmation class. Initially nominated by my classmates, it concerned me that it would be out of sympathy, not merit. However, once elected I decided to prove that I was indeed deserving of the honor.

At the confirmation service, I relished the opportunity to command the attention of a large audience. For once, I knew that people were not paying attention to me just because I was different.

During my junior and senior years, I enrolled in classes at a local Hebrew college where I earned a teaching certificate in religious education. As a student-teacher I discovered the joy of working with children, helping to shape their young minds. Of course in formulating lesson plans, I probably learned more about the subject matter than the kids! What surprised me most was just how little my disability seemed to faze the children. If anything, I commanded more respect because of it.

These kids accept me so much more easily than everyone else I'm trying to impress.

It was good to be so busy during my years in high school, as it allowed me to maintain an upbeat attitude instead of moping around feeling sorry for myself. I was involved in many of the same activities as my peers, which meant that my life didn't revolve completely around schoolwork.

But as busy as I managed to keep myself, I still experienced a great deal of emotional stress worrying what other people thought about me, even more than I had in middle school. Getting people to like me was an obsession; fitting in was more important than ever.

My disability only magnified my insecurities. I also had to contend with the need for classmates and teachers to see me like any other student. To that end I had to look, talk, and even smell just right. I even worried that the urinal in my backpack might not be clean enough and that people would think I smelled of urine! If something was hanging out of my nose, people would think I couldn't take care of myself. Combined with the intense pressure I put on myself to do well academically, it was no wonder my stomach was in knots every morning.

It also didn't help that my social life was basically nonexistent. I occasionally attended an organized event at school, a play, a dance, or a football game. Sometimes I invited a group of friends over to watch a sporting event on television. Yet the impromptu get-togethers and excursions that everyone else enjoyed were out of reach. It wasn't easy to make plans on a whim like my friends could. I wasn't able to drive, much less get into friends' cars or homes. Even if I could have gotten inside, I would have been unable to stay long due to the inevitable bathroom issues.

"Okay, everybody look the other way for a second. I'm just going to whip out my urinal and whiz into it!"

Even if my friends had considered including me in their plans, they probably realized some of the issues precluding my participation. Perhaps they felt bad about the situation and felt it was best not to invite me, although in reality I at least would have liked to have been invited.

After a while, I felt "out of sight, out of mind," attributing this mostly to the physical impracticalities imposed on me. Still, I could not help but wonder whether people liked me. Everybody was nice to me in school, but

I wondered why that never translated into my being included in their weekend plans.

Reality was that while my friends were growing more independent, I was no more independent than when I was at 12 years old. It was difficult to watch the situation unfold before my eyes, powerless to do anything about it. I envied my friends, but certainly did not begrudge them.

I wouldn't wish for them to be like me. The things they get to do, that's the way it's supposed to be.

Had I socialized more often, perhaps I would have had the confidence to ask a girl or two out on a date. I was probably just as interested in the opposite sex as the next guy, and from time to time pictured myself asking various girls if they wanted to go out. It would have involved a great deal of planning on my part and whoever went out with me would have had to understand that things might be a bit different. But I never gave myself a chance, talking myself out of the idea almost as soon as I considered it.

Why would any girl want to go out with me? I mean, I'm a decent guy, but I'm in a wheelchair. I can see past that, but would any girl be able to? Why should she?

Therefore sex wasn't considered a serious possibility. I assumed that at least some of my friends were sexually active, but simply understood that it was something for someone else, not me.

Not that I wasn't interested. Like any teenage guy, there were embarrassing moments when I was "aroused" in the presence of an attractive girl. (I only hoped no one could tell!) When it came right down to it, all I really wanted was some attention from girls.

My lack of a social life became a major source of frustration, so much so that at one point Mom and I discussed the possibility of transferring to a school in Philadelphia for students with disabilities. A few of the guys I knew with Duchenne attended school there so at least I would have known a few people. Still, I flatly rejected the option. I doubted that I would get as good an education elsewhere, as I was attending school in one of the top school districts in Pennsylvania. The whole point of going to school was to learn, not to socialize. When I felt down about my situation, I could always point to the excellent education I was receiving as justification for my lack of socializing. I wanted as normal a life as possible, and the only way I could achieve this goal was with the best education available.

Even though I often felt left out by my classmates, they were still my peers and I identified more with them than with disabled kids my age. By transferring I would have just been running away from the problem. Accepting the reality of life with a disability was my responsibility. I wasn't always going to be included and it might hurt, but it was not going to get any easier when I was out in the real world. And if I only spent time with people with disabilities, how could I gain experience interacting with "normal" people?

With transferring to a different school out of the

question, I needed to face my frustration head on. My parents arranged for me to see a psychologist. Finding someone local was not easy due to accessibility issues, but we were fortunate enough to find a local psychologist who offered to counsel me at home.

The sessions were helpful in the sense that they gave me the chance to vent my frustration even though I made a conscious effort to keep my emotions in check, fearful of crying in front of the doctor.

However, I soon realized what I already knew; there were few solutions to my problem and nothing I could do to change the reality of my situation. It was unreasonable to expect that I would not feel depressed at times. The doctor could sit there and offer his support all day, but I was going to have to get beyond my feelings because my disease was not going away anytime soon. Dad wanted to see tangible results from my sessions and often asked what I discussed with the doctor. I refused to tell him anything, citing my privacy; in reality I couldn't have pointed to any specific results even if I had tried.

I was not nearly as alone as I thought. My friends cared about me more than I knew at the time. They admired my positive attitude and constant smile. They had heard that I would be lucky to see my 21st birthday, and wondered how I could still be so upbeat. I was even the inspiration for one friend's college essay.

Friends were curious about how I spent my time outside of school. One friend tried to convince her parents to make their home accessible, while another regretted not being able to do more for me. A group of friends went as far as to pressure a school administrator into making sure I had access to the platform erected for our graduation ceremony.

With little in the way of a social life, my new-found passion for watching sports was one thing that kept me from losing my mind. Never really having played sports as a child, I didn't develop any interest in watching or discussing them. Dad had always been a big Philadelphia Eagles football fan, and on any fall Sunday afternoon I could hear him screaming at the TV during their games in a way I never heard him scream.

His interest had just never rubbed off on me. I had no idea what was so exciting about watching overweight men repeatedly run into each other.

Eventually I grew tired of feeling left out when my friends talked about their favorite teams or athletes or about games they had watched or attended. I wanted to feel as normal as they and thought that becoming a sports fan might be one way of accomplishing that goal.

Who knows, maybe it will actually be fun.

So as the NFL season began in my freshman year, I parked myself in front of the television next to Dad and watched my very first Eagles game. I watched their next game and the one after that, and before I knew it I was hooked. It was amazing how quickly I was able to learn about the game, its rules, teams, and players. Reading the sports section of the paper became a daily routine.

It was great to be able to understand what my friends

were talking about in school the next day. I think Dad also enjoyed having someone else cheer with him for the Eagles each week. When he and I had trouble finding common ground, sports was one thing we could always share.

I loved watching football so much that after getting over the Eagles' playoff loss and watching the hated Dallas Cowboys' Super Bowl victory, there was a void in my life.

Soon after I began following the other three major Philadelphia professional teams as well as local college teams. After all, watching baseball had helped me recover from spinal fusion surgery. From someone who had known next to nothing about sports, I evolved into a sports junkie. It turned out that I had an incredible capacity to remember the most obscure sports information. Fascinated by the history of teams, players, coaches and even stadiums, I developed an interest in the business side of sports and the way college and professional sports were covered by the media.

I also became hooked on sports talk radio, introduced to me by an occupational therapist who came to my home on a weekly basis. Each week, we discussed the latest sports news as he exercised my arms and legs. Then he turned on the local sports talk station, and I never looked back. I loved that it featured "guy talk" almost as often as sports talk, with hosts who discussed movies, current events, women, and personal habits. It was like having around-the-clock friends in my bedroom entertaining me, debating with me and making me laugh.

That was the real attraction of sports for me. I could

only focus on schoolwork so much, and following sports provided me with an important release. For a couple of hours I could scream my head off at the TV or radio. There was almost always something to listen to or watch. Of course if one of my teams suffered a crushing defeat, the whole idea of sports as a release for me went right out the window and I felt worse.

This sucks! I have no life. I'm stuck at home on a Saturday night watching this crap. It's really pathetic that I count on these losers to bring some joy to my life.

But my love of sports proved to be as good a replacement as possible for a social life during my high school years. Sometimes, it even created social opportunities for me when my house became the place where my friends came to watch the Super Bowl and the NCAA basketball tournament.

I was aware that they often had other plans after watching the games with me, and it was upsetting that I was never invited. But I looked at it this way: at least it was a chance to hang out with my friends. I also found that talking about sports with others was a useful icebreaker, and I used it whenever possible. People would see me as a "normal" person if they found that I had the same interests.

By the middle of my junior year, it was time to begin thinking about college. If there had ever been any doubt that I would attend college, by now it was clear that I would. Academically, there had never been any question. Though my grade point average and SAT score were not good enough to get me into an elite university, I had a decent chance at getting into many other schools.

Attending college in some far-off place was not a consideration. I wasn't sure if I could go away to school anyway. Cost was certainly a factor as well, eliminating some schools before I had a chance to look at accessibility issues.

Ultimately, my decision came down to two schools; Temple University which was about twenty minutes from home, and another school an hour away. The second school offered some scholarship money and I liked the campus, although it did not offer a true major in journalism. That was not the end of the world, but attending this school would have meant living away from home and I was going to have to feel absolutely confident that my needs could be met there from a disability standpoint.

Unfortunately when my parents and I met with the school's disability services director, I was not comfortable with her assurance that things would fall into place once I arrived as a student and that I would be able to hire student-workers to help me with personal needs.

If I couldn't find help, it was obvious that attending school there would be out of the question. It was important that I could use the toilet and get in and out of bed before I even thought about classes! It seemed a risky proposition, but I gave it great consideration. Maybe things would actually work, and I would have a chance to do something special.

How cool would it be to live away from home? I would be just like everybody else.

Initially I wasn't excited with the prospect of attending Temple, despite its reputation for disability-friendliness and a solid journalism program. It was then primarily a commuter school that someone in every Philadelphia area family had attended at one time or another.

"Temple's a good school," was the common refrain. At the time it had become common knowledge that just about anyone could get in. I had worked too hard to settle for a mediocre college education.

A visit to the university's disability services office presented concerns similar to those at the other school. The disability services coordinator assured me that while her office did not coordinate attendant care for students, they would post flyers on campus to help recruit student-workers. There it was again: student-workers. What an unsettling thought that was for me. I found it hard to believe that students were mature enough or responsible enough to be depended upon.

I can't trust people my age. And they're going to be comfortable helping me in the bathroom? I'm not even comfortable with that. I could be in a class with the same person helping me with personal stuff. They'd know all these things about me.

Attending Temple would make needing assistance with dressing, toileting, or bathing unnecessary. But even if the situation was manageable from a disability standpoint, I was still not thrilled with the school's academics.

That was until I learned about the university's honors program. With only a select number of students, it was exclusive and offered smaller classes taught by the best professors as well as extracurricular opportunities. Especially attractive was the program's personal appeal, which I had a chance to experience firsthand at an interview with one of the program's directors.

The day of my interview began inauspiciously, with a bird's dropping landing squarely on my head as my parents and I exited the parking lot! That did not do much to calm my nerves. Fortunately, the interview went much better. There were no awkward sales pitches. I had an opportunity to talk about my academic interests, the atmosphere was relaxed and the director was warm and down to earth.

Dad helped break the ice by discussing one of our favorite "historical" movies, Mel Brooks's comedic masterpiece, *History of the World, Part I*. I cited a few lines from the film and before long laughter filled the room. I came away from the interview with a favorable impression of the program and agreed to make a decision soon.

Over the next few weeks, I read correspondence from Temple, remembering how comfortable I felt with the people I met during my honors program interview. It was hard to say no. I didn't want to disappoint them; it seemed like they truly wanted me. At the same time, the opportunity to live away from home at the other school was tempting.

But truth be told, I had too many concerns about living away from home and lacked the confidence and experience at that point in my life to give it a try. Besides, it was easy to justify abandoning that opportunity, knowing how much the honors program at Temple welcomed me. And if I wanted to try living on campus at some point, it would still be possible.

Having made the decision to attend Temple, I worried that my high school classmates would be less than impressed. Sitting in my honors classes, I overheard pretentious classmates tell each other things like, "I'm going up to visit Harvard and Yale this weekend."

"So where are you looking to go, Josh?" they asked me. "Uh...Temple — Honors," I practically whispered.

You know, maybe I could have gone to one of those schools if I applied, but I have other things to think about. Okay?

The whole college shopping process was so sickening already. At least I knew where I was going, even if I was not completely thrilled about it. I had accepted my choice and was starting not to care about where anyone else was going.

By the end of senior year, I had grown more confident. Tired of deferring to others and fed up with sitting on the sidelines while everyone else seemed to be enjoying themselves, I made the decision not to let that happen anymore. It was time to be more assertive.

I asked the newspaper faculty advisor for the opportunity to write a farewell column in the final edition of the school newspaper. In previous years, I noticed that select graduating newspaper staff members had written these columns.

I wanted to address my classmates to explain why graduating with them meant so much to me. The faculty and administration had recognized my achievement with a service award, but I was not sure that my classmates understood the significance.

It turned out that writing what I wanted to get across was easier said than done. There was a fine line between pride and self-glorification that I did not want to cross.

Still, I emphasized that in all of my years as a student in the school district, I had been the only one with a disability to be mainstreamed. I could have gone elsewhere but wanted the same academic opportunities as my peers, and while I missed out socially at times it had been a necessary sacrifice.

Though accommodations had been necessary to make buildings accessible, I expressed my hope that I had proven someone with my disability could be as successful as any other student. While it had not been my primary goal, I was proud to have blazed a path for others.

Writing an article was one thing. Attending the senior prom was something entirely different. I had not attended my junior prom as I had no idea who to take, much less the courage to even ask. Attending the senior prom was a rite of passage for high school students and I was not going to miss out this time, knowing I'd regret it for the rest of my life.

Fearing a negative response, I took the plunge and

asked a girl from one of my Hebrew college classes. The words came out awkwardly.

"So, um...uh...uh...I don't know if you'd be interested, but I was wondering if you would want to go to my prom."

At 18, I had never even been on a date, so I had no experience asking this sort of thing. Before she had a chance to respond, I shot myself down as if to cushion the blow of rejection.

She's not going to want to go with me. She probably doesn't even like me. I can't look disappointed when she says no.

But she said yes—until learning the date of the prom was the same as another she had been invited to. Even so, it was as if the weight of the world had been lifted from my shoulders. I felt so much better having asked, and didn't feel the least bit discouraged that she had to say no. Now I had absolutely no idea who to ask. What I did know was that there was no way I was missing out on this prom.

One night, my sister Amy's best friend who practically lived in our house, somewhat seriously suggested that I take her. I dismissed the idea outright.

"No way! You're practically a sister to me. Amy would kill me," I chuckled.

A few days later I changed my mind. Knowing my sister's friend forever, liking her and feeling comfortable around her, was good enough. She had an outgoing personality and knew me beyond my wheelchair. I would not feel compelled to prove myself to her, and that too was appealing.

She actually wants to go with me. A girl wants to go out with me and I'm going to turn her down? This never happens. I can't say no!

My heart raced as I dialed her phone number a few days later. She said yes and I was thrilled. Everything was perfect, until I found out the night before the prom that my date was sick with a high fever. My heart sank, but I felt worse for her, not wanting her to feel guilty for being unable to go with me.

Fortunately, her condition improved just enough by the next day. When her mom brought her over to our house, I couldn't believe how stunning she looked. It was like I was in a dream. I didn't get to go out with pretty girls; that was someone else's life.

Fittingly dressed in a tuxedo for the occasion, excitement was in the air as Dad chauffeured us to the historic downtown hotel where the prom was held. Once there, I was too nervous to eat and my date was too sick, which made the situation a bit awkward. Concerned with how my date was feeling I felt guilty that she had pushed herself for me, but most of all felt angry that we had been seated at a table in an inaccessible location with people I hardly knew.

The loser table. Just great. And I wonder why I never go to events like this.

But I was determined to have a good time anyway. We decided to venture onto the dance floor and found a way to "dance" as my pretty date placed her hands on my shoulders and we moved back and forth together. I thought this might look strange to other people, but for once I didn't care what they thought. I felt normal. It was a huge step for me.

The next day, I woke up with an emotional hangover. My first date was an accomplishment in the sense that I had finally been able to do something everybody else did. And yet, I was so depressed. After all of the build-up, it was over.

I've waited to do something like this the entire time I was in high school. Why didn't I do it sooner?

My emotions about graduating from high school were even more mixed. Academically, it was a stepping stone and nothing more. There was much more to accomplish. I had fully expected to complete high school, even if my family wondered about that when I was diagnosed with muscular dystrophy nearly fourteen years earlier. I was proud to have been mainstreamed throughout my entire education, the only student in the school district to do so.

Except when it was time to graduate, I was not the only student in a wheelchair. It turned out that another student from the township was entitled to graduate with our class even though he had attended a school for disabled students. Though I kept my thoughts to myself, I was concerned that people would think, "How wonderful. Two kids in wheelchairs were able to achieve like everyone else."

I'm the one who deserves the credit. Buildings had to be made accessible on account of me. I was here from the start.

Not going out of my way to welcome him during graduation rehearsals I tried to be cordial, knowing him from camp and figuring he didn't know anyone other than me. Still, I was afraid of what everyone else would think.

They're automatically going to assume we're friends just because we're both in wheelchairs. I have so much more in common with everyone else.

With the excitement of graduation night, it no longer mattered. Receiving a standing ovation as I drove across the podium to accept my diploma, I blushed with embarrassment at being singled out. Realizing that people respected my accomplishment was incredibly satisfying. Graduation went by much too quickly. After celebrating with my family late into the night, I had to get up early the next morning for college orientation.

Though I would have preferred going to orientation by myself, I needed someone to drive me in addition to assist me in the bathroom and with lunch. My grandfather agreed to accompany me, but he kept a low profile, so it wasn't too bad—until it was time for the safe sex presentation!

Like that's ever going to be an issue for me anyway.

Even so, watching how to put a rubber on a banana with my grandfather was just a bit awkward. I turned to him, sheepishly asking, "You sure you're old enough to be hearing this?"

By the end of orientation, I couldn't wait for the first semester to begin. I felt strong, healthy and motivated.

There was much to accomplish and the sky was the limit. Nothing was going to stop me now.

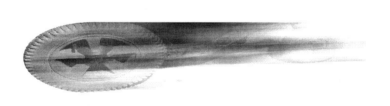

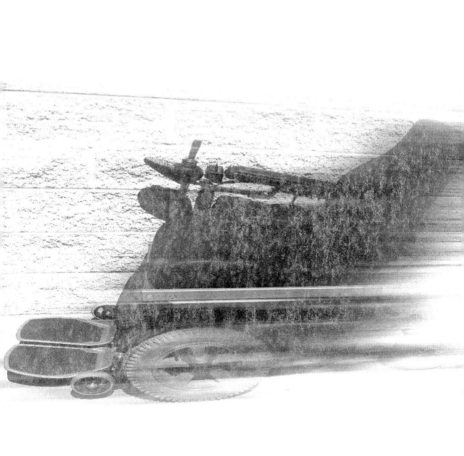

After exactly two days on the job, the first attendant I ever hired disappeared off the face of the earth. That was, until pay day when she called to say she wanted to stop by to pick up her check (which couldn't have been more than $15) and to inform us she was quitting. Big surprise, not that I would have wanted her to come back after she showed up to retrieve her check looking like a drug addict.

I couldn't imagine how someone could quit so soon. In her time on the job, she had not done so much as lift a finger. All she did was observe Mom, who demonstrated how to help me.

It was not a good start to my experience with attendant care services. Everything had sounded so simple when I met the caseworker from the agency who had been contracted by the state to provide attendant care services. Based on the amount of time it took to complete tasks such as eating, brushing my teeth, toileting, bathing, and getting dressed, I qualified for three hours of care divided equally in the morning and at night. Although the agency was responsible for paying attendants and could help me recruit and screen them, I had the hiring and firing power.

I had grown accustomed to Mom providing all of my care, and was less than amenable to having someone else do the job. The only extended period of time during which someone else provided my care was at summer camp. I needed much less help then, but still hated the experience.

Now 18 years old, I wanted to become more independent, which meant needing Mom less. Sure, I would still be dependent on someone else, but they would be hired by me and I would be the one to tell them what was needed.

Unfortunately, I soon found that many attendants behaved exactly the same way my first attendant did. Getting people to consistently show up for work was half the battle regardless of what I said to the potential attendants during interviews.

"I need you to be on time, but call me if you are running late. If you're not going to be able to make it, I expect you to let me know ahead of time. I understand that things happen. If something comes up suddenly, call me."

So they understood my need to stress these rules, I described some of my previous problems with unreliable attendants. If I had a dollar for every time a person said, "I can't believe people do that to you. That's just not right. I'm not like that," I would have become a millionaire.

Having someone in my home to take care of me required an adjustment period which was repeated every time a new attendant was hired. The whole concept of meeting a total stranger one minute and having that person see me naked or wipe my ass the next was just a bit unnerving. I was an extremely private person and didn't like sharing my bodily functions with someone else!

When someone new was working for me, it took time to feel comfortable going to the bathroom with that person next door. After a while I grew less self-conscious, comforted by the knowledge that my attendants considered what they did for me routine.

This is what she does. It's not like she's never wiped someone's ass before.

The process of training an attendant was nerve wracking. With Mom demonstrating, I taught new recruits how to use the Hoyer lift without dropping the chains on me or banging my knees when moving me. From carefully dressing me, to helping me with the urinal without spilling it on me, to positioning the pillows on the bed to support my legs, we covered every conceivable detail of my care.

But each time a new attendant started, I was nervous that he or she would injure me since my bones were fragile and my limbs contracted. Telling someone my legs could not be extended was one thing; proving it was another.

How many times do I have to say not to stretch my leg!

"Uh, you're stretching my leg too far. That hurts," I would gently remind the attendant.

Some people were more heavy-handed than others. Putting on a pair of socks could be a real adventure with some due to my sensitive toes, while others could be so cautious that it took forever to complete tasks like sliding my pants off.

I eased attendants into the job by initially limiting their tasks. One night I had the person bathe me, the next time I had he or she take me to the toilet and then put me in bed. This way there was plenty of time, making sure the person didn't feel rushed. And I didn't lose my mind!

The better attendants picked up my routine more easily, but few were as efficient as Mom who had years of practice. I knew that having someone else help was important to my sense of independence and to Mom who deserved a break. Still, training new attendants took time and patience.

How do I tell her she's an idiot without actually calling her an idiot?

I quickly learned that most people did not take too kindly to criticism, and worried that if I came across overly critical they might take their frustration out on me.

I learned to correct people in a calm voice, reminding myself that no one was perfect and that mistakes were bound to occur. Of course it only took one slip-up for me to get hurt, which happened from time to time. I repeated the same instructions over and over, trying never to appear frustrated even if my blood was boiling inside. I also tried to bite my tongue when experiencing slight pain while being bathed or moved, figuring that no one liked a complainer.

Displaying such patience, I was not about to tolerate being intimidated in my own home. One night, I gently reminded an attendant who was over-aggressively putting my arm into a shirt that she needed to be more careful. "I have a baby. I know how to be careful," she said.

Not exactly. And I'm not a baby!

That kind of attitude was not acceptable. My physical limitations made me essentially helpless, but I was also someone's "boss" as much as I disliked the term, and didn't want to be pushed around by someone working for me.

To their credit, most of my attendants were able to look beyond my disability and respect me. It made me wonder why the rest of the world couldn't treat people with disabilities the same way.

In return, I met my obligations to the attendants, submitting their timesheets on time and ensuring that they had a chance to work at least the number of hours we had agreed upon. If I didn't need help one night, it was unfair to penalize my attendant. However, the only legitimate option was to allow him to make up the hours another night, which was obviously less convenient for the attendant than had I not cancelled in the first place.

I learned how to communicate effectively, and heard some horror stories about clients who were racist, dictatorial, unreasonable, arbitrary, or downright hostile. No one wanted to work for someone like that. The trick was to be firm without being mean, to be specific but not demanding. I never raised my voice (even though it probably would have felt great at times) and was uncomfortable being forceful when giving instructions. I was willing to consider suggestions from my attendants, but in the long run things had to be done my way. I often prefaced my directions with phrases like "Would you mind..." or said something like, "Should we shave my face next?"

I'm not really asking your opinion; what I mean is, "Do it."

Another tack I took was to poke fun at myself. "I know you probably think it's a stupid thing, but..." I said.

If I or someone in my family had any concerns about an attendant, it was my responsibility to handle the situation. Though I was living in their house, my parents expected me to take charge.

"They're your employees," Dad was quick to remind me. Of course, that never stopped him from complaining. "She's too loud. He's on the phone too much. She's always calling out of work. He's never on time," he would point out.

Sometimes I agreed; other times, I did not. If something needed to be said, I was going to be the one to say it. Never the confrontational type, problems often festered. I was afraid to rush to judgment as that always seemed to backfire, and was hesitant to say things out of fear of losing attendants. This would only have meant more work for Mom while I searched for someone new.

For the most part I got along well with my attendants, and believed they liked working for me because I was fair and grateful for their help. I also tried to do small favors for them. If they needed to use my phone, it was no problem; if they wanted to watch TV while I was in the bathroom, it was fine. I gave them clothes I no longer wore, and if it was someone's birthday in my house my attendant got a piece of cake. I asked about their lives and listened patiently to their problems, even when I was bored or tired. My hope was that by treating people well, they would want to do a better job.

Perhaps it was self-serving, but being nice did not require a concerted effort on my part. Even if attendants were paid to be there, I still considered them guests in my house. On a subconscious level I wanted everyone to be my friend, even if that was not ideal in an employer-employee relationship.

This was not a typical business relationship, unlike that of an office job where the boss instructs employees and they go their separate ways. An attendant's job was much more personal. He or she interacted with one person the entire shift. It was more comfortable when both parties liked each other.

Most of the attendants seemed to appreciate my kindness. They picked up items at the store for me, cooked homemade food for me, gave me gifts at the holidays, and brought their children to meet me.

Unfortunately, it was hard to count on most attendants for more than a few months. It was frustrating to invest my time training an attendant, only to have to replace that person. The process of getting comfortable with someone new would just have to be repeated. It was also difficult in the sense that I often grew attached to my attendants. I saw the good in them and had a hard time understanding why they had suddenly become so unreliable. This served to remind me that at the end of the day, it was a job. There was nothing wrong with growing close to someone, but if he or she was not living up to their end of the bargain, then it was time to cut the cord.

Not that it was easy to fire attendants; I was taking away from their livelihood, which made me feel guilty. It also put me in a vulnerable position because I could never predict how they would react to my decision.

I was never able to say, "You're fired" but found ways to get the message across. Many times it was simply understood. The person never showed up again and never called.

Once, I was so enraged that I left a strongly-worded message on an attendant's cell phone. I held back from cursing her out, but nonetheless gave her a piece of my mind.

"I cannot believe you're doing this to me. I am very disappointed. It's not like I haven't given you chance after chance. You have made me look like a fool. And you don't even have the decency to return my phone calls," I said in a surprisingly calm tone.

Whenever I was between attendants Mom took care of me; at times this lasted as long as a few months. It was easy to get comfortable with this arrangement. After all, Mom was the most efficient "attendant" around.

When I became busy with my college career, it was nice not to adhere to the set hours of an attendant. Mom and I both enjoyed not having to worry whether or not someone was going to show up. Still, it was not the ideal situation in the long run.

Just when my search for new attendants reached rock bottom, I found a candidate who restored my faith in the system. When he called for an interview I was highly skeptical, having grown weary of hiring and firing attendants. As we talked at the kitchen table, I immediately liked the guy. He had an outgoing, upbeat but calm demeanor. We talked about sports and he laughed at my sense of humor. Being a nice guy was one thing. But would he be serious enough?

My question was answered when I learned that his experience came from caring for his granddad who had a serious illness. He explained that he had taken on this responsibility because he was worried about how hired caregivers treated his granddad.

Not only did he prove trustworthy, but he had an easy-going, fun personality. It was never a chore to have him around. And when it was time to get to work, to dress me, wash me or anything else, he was careful, thorough, and efficient.

That is, except when he gave me a shower. As he scrubbed me from head to toe, we talked up a storm, oblivious to the time that lapsed and the amount of water we wasted.

As time went by, he became an extended member of the family. Dad and he talked about bargains at clothing outlet stores. (In fact, he had such good taste in clothes that I had him choose my attire each day.) Mom chatted with him about his girlfriend and infant daughter. He even served as a "bouncer" at Amy's 16th birthday party!

For me, it was like having a new friend. At night after putting me in bed, he and I played video games or got "on the sticks" as he called it. If he saw me as his employer, he certainly did not show it as he beat me up and down the court, rink or field!

Unfortunately though, it was still a working relationship and reliability became a major issue. Often, I called him a half hour after he was supposed to be at my house.

"Where are you?" I asked. "I'm on my way. I got stuck working at my uncle's store, but I'll be there," he assured me. Eventually he arrived, sometimes as much as an hour later.

Mornings were also interesting. My usual 6 A.M. wakeup time was normally manageable for him, but days that I had a later class and could sleep in a bit were not. This was ostensibly because after a night out he had a chance to go home and fall asleep. He didn't have that chance when I needed him at 6 A.M.

Uncomfortable as it was for me to do I tried confronting him on his lack of reliability, which had little effect on the problem. Finally, I had no choice but to fire him. It was difficult to do, but I had put it off long enough. Now was the time to be an adult and do what was necessary. At the same time, this was no joke. My decision would have a serious impact on my attendant's life and I knew it.

Who else my age has this kind of responsibility?

"Look, you know I like having you here. Everyone in my family does. You are the best attendant I've ever had and I hate to lose you," I explained.

He reacted about as well as I could have expected. I knew he was disappointed, but he admitted that I had been fair and that he understood my decision.

I was glad we remained friendly. He even returned to work for me briefly, and a couple of years later he was there for my college graduation party.

A number of other memorable attendants worked for me as time went on. They came to work for various reasons. Some wanted a few hours of work while they stayed home with their children; others wanted to supplement their income from full-time office jobs. Some cobbled four or five attendant jobs together to make some semblance of a living; others simply liked helping people.

My favorite attendants had varying personalities. Some were very businesslike, in and out the door. Others were more laid back; they let me lay in bed for a few extra minutes while chatting with my family. All were pleasant, personable and hard-working.

Overall however, good attendants were not always easy to find, which I attributed to the poor compensation they received. Simply saying that if someone takes a job she's supposed to be there on time and ready to work did nothing to solve the problem.

After all, how many people were interested in working for nine dollars an hour for an hour and half? Combined with the fact that many attendants lived in the city and relied on public transportation, there was good reason why some people were less than committed to their jobs.

These were circumstances beyond my control. All I could do was hire the best people I could find and cross my fingers. I had a life to live and there were better things for me to do than worry about who was going to wipe my ass that night!

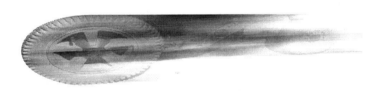

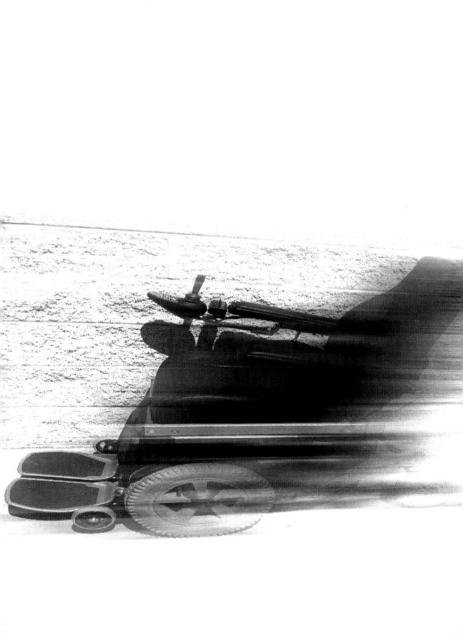

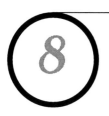

On my first day of college, I did what any other mature 18-year-old did in the face of adversity: I cried.

"I can't do this. It's too much," I sobbed, as I told Mom about my day.

After a full day of classes and an hour in line at the campus bookstore, my paratransit ride home had been an hour and a half late. Three or four phone calls to the dispatch center were useless, but I had tried to remain calm.

When the inexperienced and overwhelmed driver arrived, I was tired but cordial. It took him forever to secure my wheelchair to the vehicle, and when the straps came loose a few blocks from campus I had to ask him to pull over and tighten them. He insisted the straps were tight, although they clearly were not.

Fighting rush-hour traffic, we managed to get halfway to my house when the dispatch center called, instructing the driver to turn around and go in the complete opposite direction downtown for another pickup. That was the end of my patience. Enraged, I could no longer hold my tongue.

"You tell him there's no fucking way!" I shouted at the top of my lungs, "Do you know how late you were? We're almost at my house and now you're going to turn around? That's crazy!"

I lost my argument. At 7 P.M. I arrived home, three hours after my scheduled pickup time, exhausted, stressed, hungry, and needing to pee desperately.

In between my tears, I realized that my plan to spend time every day on campus after classes so I could get involved socially was not practical. This was only the beginning of my trials and tribulations with paratransit or "parastranded" as it was known by many in the disabled community! With all the time and energy it took from me, it was almost like taking an extra class each semester.

Sometimes, I was picked up and taken to the other side of town for another pickup, what I called "the city tour."

If you don't drive fast, my bladder's going to burst!

Other times, the drivers got lost. "Yeah, the driver is right outside your house," I got a call.

"Uh, I'm outside my house and I don't see him," I said, incredulously, "The driver does realize that I'm located in Montgomery County, not Philadelphia? Because there's a street with the same name in Philly..."

There were times when everything was going just fine and suddenly something absolutely ridiculous would happen. Like the time we were riding up a hill and the poorly-maintained vehicle's transmission gave out. Or the time a safety latch broke, preventing the vehicle from starting, which was also necessary to operate the lift!

The biggest issue was lateness. As it was so hard to count on their timeliness, I scheduled rides allowing three times the amount of time it took to get from home to campus, just to "cover my ass." Often that wasn't even enough time.

As a result I was always on edge, my stomach was in knots, and I got a sinking feeling if my ride was even five minutes late. There was nothing worse than finishing up a long, exhausting day only to wait another hour for a ride. It didn't make the prospect of spending the night reading textbooks any better.

I was often frustrated but hardly kept quiet, demanding accountability. "Look, if you were late for work every day, you wouldn't have a job," I tried to reason with customer service representatives. "My professors don't care that I'm in a wheelchair, and they shouldn't. They expect me to be on time."

I even was adamant that a statement be written to a professor to whose class I arrived chronically late. "It's not a big deal; you don't need to do that," he assured me.

"No, no. There's no reason they can't get me here on time when they've been given 90 minutes for a 25-minute ride," I insisted.

Sometimes I was able to secure vouchers for complimentary rides, although once I was asked to pay $1 along with the coupon. "But it says 'complimentary,' not 'partially complimentary,'" I protested.

There was one particular occasion I did regret opening my mouth. That was after the driver got lost and never showed up, causing me to miss an Eagles game. After multiple calls to the dispatcher that day, I was in tears. The only consolation was the Eagles lost, 30-0. Still, having blown $90 on game tickets, I contacted the owner of the paratransit company demanding compensation for my loss.

Instead he offered to take Mom and me to see a Temple football game in his box seats, transportation provided by one of his best drivers. I knew it was going to be an interesting day as we boarded the vehicle that morning to find the driver's strung-out girlfriend in one of the seats. About 20 minutes later we passed the airport.

"Uh, I thought the stadium was *before* the airport...," I spoke up. We would have wound up in another state if I hadn't opened my mouth.

When we finally arrived, we were aggravated and starving. Problem was the idiot owner had forgotten to order food! Soon we were watching the god-awful Temple Owls get annihilated, gobbling down cold hot dogs and listening to the owner talk about wanting to fire the obnoxious dispatcher who actually arrived at the game moments later. I couldn't wait to go home, wishing to have my $90 instead.

One thing I learned dealing with paratransit was that the drivers who were given unreasonable schedules that never took into account the traffic or the time it took to secure wheelchairs, were rarely at fault. In fact, I became friendly with several drivers, often talking with them about sports, but sometimes the conversation shifted to poverty, racism or politics. I enjoyed hearing opinions different from those shaped by my upbringing. Sometimes, we became so engrossed in conversation that the driver forgot where he was going.

"Hey, uh, Al, you just passed my house!" We both laughed hysterically as he put the vehicle in reverse.

There were also some incredibly belligerent drivers, like the one I warned to be careful as he leaned over me to secure my wheelchair. "My bones break easily," I explained.

"What's the difference? You're already broken," he sneered.

No you didn't!

"Excuse me! I am NOT! You are! I can't believe you just said that," I lashed back.

I ratted him out the next day, although I was initially hesitant to call the company because dispatch was sometimes dumb enough to send drivers back who I had complained about in the past.

That driver notwithstanding, I wasn't about to let paratransit break me in any sense of the word. I was going places and nothing was going to stop me.

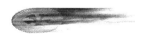

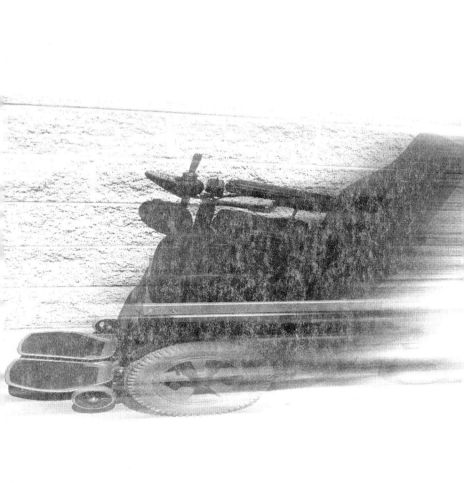

The Time of My Life

9

Parastranded or not, there was no way I was going to let my transportation issues get in the way of my education. A few weeks into my first semester, any doubts I had about my college choice were erased. I couldn't imagine how my education might have been better at a pricier or more prestigious university. In my view, the education I received was only as strong as the effort I put forth. And I did just that, with great success.

Though continuing to excel in the liberal arts as in high school, I wanted to prove I could be successful in any area as long as I was willing to put forth the effort. Having inadvertently registered for a challenging math class, I decided to stick with it anyway just to prove to myself that I was not a one-dimensional student. I studied hard and spent every other day in the professor's office for additional help.

Overall, most of my classes were enjoyable as were

the professors who taught them. I became most passionate about the courses in my American studies minor, which combined American history, politics, and culture. I took a course on immigration that awakened me to the struggles and sacrifices of previous generations, and helped me better understand the newest immigrants.

A course on radicalism allowed me to form a different view of socialism and communism, while another course focused on the tumultuous 1960s and how they changed society. All of the courses examined the American experience from the perspective of the disenfranchised. As a result I realized that despite my disease and personal struggles, I was still more fortunate than many Americans.

Although I was fairly healthy, my good health wasn't going to last indefinitely so I felt it was essential to graduate on time. For this reason, I took five classes each semester. The problem was that my transportation situation limited the amount of time I could spend on campus, which left time for only four classes.

To remedy the situation I often took courses during the summer semesters; during the regular year I took online courses in addition to those on campus. With my disability, online courses offered some benefits. I could work at my own pace; if I needed to take a break, I could do so. I didn't have to worry about taking notes, and could participate in class e-mail "discussions" without signaling the professor to let him know I wanted to speak. Eventually I lost my ability to type, which made things a bit more challenging, but online courses proved quite helpful.

Generally speaking, attending college was easy from a disability standpoint. Temple's disabilities office, with several hundred registered students who had physical and learning disabilities, had a system in place. At the beginning of each semester, the office prepared letters I presented to professors that outlined the accommodations approved for me. In my case, such accommodations included the use of a tape recorder and the presence of an attendant in class. Although I was able to write, it now took longer, so I was allowed double time for exams, which were administered at the disabilities office's testing center.

This system encouraged disabled students to take initiative in discussing their needs with professors. Admittedly, I was at an advantage. The fact that I was in a wheelchair confirmed my disability. At the same time, I looked normal otherwise, didn't have embarrassing facial tics or anything else unusual and therefore was confident approaching someone new. More importantly, I could speak normally. As a result it was easier for professors who encountered me, as opposed to some of the other students with disabilities. Just as I was growing as a person with a disability, having students with disabilities was a learning experience for even the most considerate professors. One of my favorite professors agreed that during class discussions, she would call on me when I pointed my pen. A few weeks later, she wondered why I had been so quiet in class.

"You never look to your right, and that's where I sit," I explained.

Simply because a system was in place did not mean that it had all the answers. Sometimes a bit of creativity was necessary, as in the case of the copy editing course I was required to take one semester. Taught by a busy editor at the *Philadelphia Inquirer,* the class began at 8:10 in the morning and was the only section of the class offered. There was simply no way I could count on paratransit to get me there at that hour.

I didn't see an easy fix, but after discussions between the instructor and the director of disability services an unusual solution was found. I would "attend" class by speakerphone, listening to class lectures from my bedroom. It proved to be an excellent idea, and it showed what was possible even without any legal maneuvering when people were willing to think outside of the box. Still, it was my job to justify the effort made on my behalf. So at precisely 8:10 A.M. I dialed into class and worked as hard as my virtual classmates.

Temple's disability resources office didn't address my biggest concern from an accessibility standpoint. Who was going to help me on campus? The office neither recruited nor paid attendants, which was somewhat puzzling. The way I figured, being able to eat or go to the bathroom was more important than extended time for tests. Without a way of taking care of these basic needs, college was anything but accessible.

Finding an attendant for my freshman year was a

challenge; with only a few weeks before the semester began, I had no real leads from a flyer posted on campus. Fortunately, another guy with Duchenne who I had gotten to know over the years had found an attendant, a man he met through his church. He offered to share his attendant, who was also in school and happy to earn a few extra dollars. I immediately said yes.

Pennsylvania's Office of Vocational Rehabilitation (OVR) which helped people with disabilities become employable, agreed to pay my attendant $5 an hour. It was a measly sum, but the "thirty-something" father of several children didn't seem to mind. His wife had a full-time job and he said he liked helping people.

I was grateful for this man's assistance, which made my transition to college much less worrisome. I settled into a familiar routine. He sat with me in classes during which I needed to shuffle books and papers. For other classes, my attendant would set me up and return when the class was over. When I had to go to the bathroom he was not squeamish about the fact that I now required help putting my penis into the urinal, which was a great relief to me.

When it was time for lunch, he helped me purchase my food and carry it back to the disabilities office. I needed help un-wrapping a sandwich and placing it in my hand, but I could feed myself by placing a soda can on my wheelchair tray, resting my hand on the can, and leaning down to reach the food in my hand.

I spent a good portion of the day with my attendant

during which we both enjoyed a nice time. We were always talking about something, from the then-wretched Eagles, to pretty girls; from strange professors, to politics and religion. (I assured him I had no intention of converting from Judaism!)

My attendant also initially helped me "break the ice" with my classmates. He was extremely outgoing and they liked talking to him. His presence made it easier for people to approach and talk to me. At times, he attempted to steer conversations he had with my classmates toward me, which was helpful.

For my first year and a half of college, I was content to focus on my studies. But something wasn't right. While I was getting a quality education, it didn't seem that I was taking advantage of the entire college experience.

College was supposed to be about more than hitting the books. I had participated in few activities and spent most of my time hanging out with my attendant rather than with friends. I had little more than two years left and it would all be over. And what would I really have, aside from a piece of paper?

Determined not to let the rest of my college years slip away, it was time to take control of my life. I started by firing my attendant whose presence had initially been reassuring, but had become a major liability. He was rarely on time and often moody, similar to the grumpy man who helped me in high school.

Why do I have to put up with this crap? I'm not always

in a good mood, but I never take it out on the people who help me. I always act professionally. Why can't he?

It was a waste to have him in class with me because I didn't need all that much help, and I was overshadowed by his presence as classmates talked to him before me. Encouraged by professors to participate in class, he made stupid points that I felt reflected negatively on me. Worse yet, I suspected him of stealing from me. After giving him my wallet to purchase my lunch, I often found the wallet lighter and his hands filled with several items for himself. It was probably an offense for which I should have fired him immediately, but I had no specific proof.

Even so, I never accused him of any wrongdoing and felt bad about putting a person out of work. Moreover, it seemed like replacing him would be more trouble than it was worth, so I kept trying to justify keeping him.

Is he that bad? Sure, he's not as reliable as I'd like, and maybe he's not that pleasant. But I know what to expect from him. Do I really need the stress of finding someone else?

After agonizing for weeks, I simply explained to him that it was time for me to become more independent. And that was no lie. He had been a safety net for me, but I needed to grow up and depend on myself. Still, finding the right words was difficult. I was much more diplomatic in those days. As classmates and professors asked about him, I took the high road. "We've sort of parted ways," I told them.

There were many things that people saw about me,

but I needed to keep certain things behind closed doors to feel I had some control over my life.

But who would help me? I still needed someone to help me get lunch, use the bathroom, and sometimes walk with me to class and help me set up. Initially, I considered asking friends because I thought they would be more familiar and more reliable. However, I worried that everyone I met would become someone to take care of me. Furthermore, most of my friends were girls, which sounded good at first. But would they be comfortable helping me in the bathroom?

In the end, I decided I would feel more comfortable hiring people I didn't know. Skeptical that I would find anyone, I requested that the disabilities office post flyers on campus. Much to my surprise, I received three or four responses to my ad within a few days.

Hiring students turned out to be a great arrangement. The students I chose to help me were usually very responsible, which I attributed to the fact that most Temple students were working their way through college. If they were not serious, their education could have been seriously jeopardized.

I also had the opportunity to meet all types of people. I hired a veritable United Nations of Indians, Koreans, African-Americans, and Hispanics. The countless philosophical discussions over lunch about popular culture, religion, and politics were enlightening. A few of the students even became good friends. Such friendships were unique in the sense that they had helped me with personal things in the past, so I was comfortable asking them to help me with the urinal, whereas I never would have asked my other friends.

I did hire some female students to assist me at the times I typically did not use the bathroom. One time, I needed to go to the bathroom and had no choice. A pretty lacrosse player was assisting me. Though she assured me in the past that she didn't mind, she became squeamish about touching me.

"I don't want to hurt you; I don't have much experience with [penises]," she told me.

Just great. She's a virgin. But I really have to go. Besides, it's not like I'm a pervert; I'm a virgin, too. And she's wearing latex gloves, so I couldn't enjoy her touching me even if I wanted to!

The "kick in the pants" I received from an advisor at the disability services office also helped me take control of my life. When I was lamenting one day to her about my wheelchair's propensity to suddenly die in the middle of the street, she responded by implying that I was using the situation as an excuse, even if it had some legitimacy.

"Just go out there. You'll be fine," she said.

"But what if my wheelchair stops in the middle of the street?" I asked.

"So ask someone to cross the street with you," was her answer.

Well, I guess that might work. No decent person's going to leave me.

I had been so concerned about the problem that I failed to think of such a simple solution. And so I began venturing out on campus myself. What a liberating feeling!

I got too brave one frigid morning when no one was around and I was in a hurry to cross Broad Street, Philadelphia's main north-south route. Because the subway ran beneath it, the street had a pronounced crown. As I neared the middle of the road, my cold hand slipped off my joystick and I could not move.

Don't panic. It's not like the light's green and you're in the middle of the busiest street in the city. Wait, it is and I am!

Fortunately a quick-thinking bus driver noticed me, jumped out of his bus and bolted across the street. I told him how to disengage the motors and he pushed me to safety. My heart left my throat and I took a deep breath.

I learned my lesson, but continued to embrace my new-found independence. If I didn't panic, there was always a solution. I just had to figure it out.

On an afternoon when one of my helpers called out sick and I had eaten nothing all day, I had a half-hour to spare before my ride home. I could have waited, but I was hungry. I asked the secretary in the disabilities office to place my wallet on my wheelchair tray, and headed to a hot dog cart where I asked for a canned drink. Placing my hand on the can, I asked the vendor to put the sandwich in my other hand. I leaned over and chowed down on my lunch. Then matter-of-factly I drove around the corner to wait for my ride.

Just doing what any normal person would do. No help? No problem.

Pretty soon, my new-found confidence had spread to other areas. I tried new things and jumped at opportunities, like getting a job as a student writer at the university's communications office. When I responded to a request from the office for students to be interviewed by a local newspaper, I was offered the position.

"Are you calling about the e-mail or for the job?" asked the staff writer who answered.

"Uh..." I hesitated.

What the hell am I doing? What's the worst that could happen?

"...Both?" I answered nervously.

My assignments consisted mostly of writing boilerplate press releases and photo captions, usually to let students' hometown newspapers know when they won awards. I also had a chance to do some interviews and write some longer articles. I learned about large developments on campus and who the bigwigs were at the university. Whatever the task, I performed it like it was the most important job in the world.

I was still able to type and use a mouse, so I simply asked the secretaries to place the keyboard and mouse on my wheelchair tray; I also needed some help retrieving files. The only real accommodation necessary was a headset telephone for making calls. Initially, I felt bad that I was a part-time student worker and they were going to spend part of their budget for me. Even if they were required by law to accommodate me, I felt the need to justify an expense like that by doing my very best. From day one, I felt the need to prove myself to the staff. Besides demonstrating that I was a good writer, I had to prove that someone with a disability could do the job. To their credit, the staff recognized my ability off the bat and my physical limitations became a non-issue. They regarded me as one of the best student writers ever, but some of the staff members grew concerned with how I was feeling physically. At times, I didn't feel my best, but it was important to show up and do a good job anyway because that was what people did. I was not about to use my disability as an excuse. Once that was established, becoming friendly with the staff and feeling comfortable engaging in the sort of water cooler talk that was a part of office culture seemed natural.

A few months later, I added another job tutoring students taking a university-mandated literature survey course. I was confident that I was qualified, knowing the material and how to write. Learning to tutor students was a different story. It required balancing encouragement and constructive criticism, and it turned out that I was well-suited for the job. It was nice that instead of people helping me, I was helping them for a change.

In addition to my two jobs I also began writing for the *Temple News,* the campus newspaper. I started slowly writing minor pieces that I knew would be easy and not very time consuming. Eventually, I had the opportunity to write more important articles: a profile about the disabilities office, an article about the university's acquisition of a new school, a front-page story about a dispute between a neighborhood athletic organization and the university.

As in high school, I took great pride in my writing and being one of the most reliable staff writers. Because the students who served as my editors were also classmates from the journalism program, I actually felt little need to prove that I could be reliable despite my disability. One editor (and friend) knew that unlike other writers, she never had to worry about stories she assigned to me. She was confident that I only took on what I could handle and that she could to count on getting "good, clean copy." I never sought to be an editor at the paper, though I was confident that I could have handled such a position. There was simply too much on my plate and not enough time.

Now, I was beginning to realize my potential as a college student. Apparently, people around me began to notice as well. They saw me as a leader. The staff at the disabilities office used me as an example to other students with disabilities because I had been able to get involved on campus instead of making the office my home base.

Most importantly, I was recognized as a leader beyond my disability. I was proud to be invited to speak on behalf of the entire student body at a ceremony honoring the university's top faculty members. Another tremendous honor was being selected as the sole student representative on a committee tasked with choosing a new dean for the school of communications. This allowed me the opportunity to interact with high-ranking university officials. My advisor had nominated me because she believed I was a student with integrity. However, little did she and some of my professors know how tight-lipped I would be when they tried to "pump" me for details about the search process!

With each achievement, I gained more and more confidence in my abilities. I was no longer concerned if I gained attention because of my disability. If it got me in the door, fine. Given time, I would make a believer out of everyone. My thought was that if people had their eyes on me, I would turn it into something positive.

Five classes, two jobs, newspaper assignments, in addition to transportation and attendant care issues raised my stress level. Yet I was never happier. I was not living the life of a person with a disease, but the life of a "normal" person. Completely occupied with my routine, I didn't have time to think about my disease.

Though probably hurting my health down the road, I lived my life full speed ahead, pushing my body even when I was exhausted. I had little choice. While other people had the rest of their lives ahead of them with families and careers, I didn't have the luxury of time and needed to take advantage of every opportunity. Fortunately, the university setting was a microcosm of the outside world, and offered me the chance to try many things.

Riding home from classes one beautiful fall afternoon, it became apparent just how fortunate I was. With the combination of maturity and stable health, I knew my life might never be better.

I need to enjoy this while it lasts. It's not going to last forever. It's only a matter of time before things get worse.

I had seen the future and it did not look good. At a party hosted by my friends and fellow Duchenne patients, Brian and Michael, I saw some of the first guys who were on ventilators and had tracheotomies. It looked like a highly unpleasant existence. They seemed rather quiet, especially in comparison to the loud machines used to suction mucous from their trachs, seemingly every other minute.

"A trach is the last thing they do to you before you die," one of the other guys at the party said to me. "I'd rather just die when I need one."

I felt the same way at the time, and also never wanted to spend time with those guys again; it was just too depressing.

Compared to my high school years, I was slightly more successful from a social standpoint. One reason was that in addition to courses, the honors program offered numerous organized events, field trips and other social gatherings. Such activities offered unique opportunities to interact with fellow students, and because they were planned in advance, I was usually able to make arrangements to attend.

During a trip to Washington, D.C., I had a chance to get to know my classmates away from the classroom, and they had a glimpse into my life — from riding in an accessible bus, to watching me get accosted by a crazed veteran at the Vietnam War Memorial.

On the way, I opened up to a few of my classmates about some of the realities of my disease.

"If I hurt my arm, I might stop moving it for a while and pretty soon I could lose that ability," I explained.

I had always tried to avoid making my disability the focus, but it felt so good to know that people actually cared about what my life was like.

Advisors and professors went out of their way to make sure events were accessible to me. When a professor held a party at her historic home, I had some obvious accessibility concerns but agreed to attend. Behind the scenes, an advisor, in consultation with the disabilities office, obtained a portable ramp. At another event on campus, an elevator was not working so the director and three students carried me up a flight of stairs in my wheelchair, some 300 pounds.

Sometimes, I had to rely on friends to help so I could attend an event. When invited to sit in box seats at a basketball game as part of a contingent of honors students, I was unable to find an assistant. I was not going to have a chance to eat before the game but food would be available there. I would need to ask someone for help but was afraid of being even the slightest burden to people I liked.

Just because people are my friends doesn't mean they should have to be responsible for me.

"There won't be anyone to help me, so I was wondering if you'd mind getting my food with me," I said to a friend on the phone the night before, "If there's food that needs to be cut, I might need some help with that, too."

Whatever the event, I always took the initiative by checking into accessibility and transportation. It was something Mom had instilled in me over the years. Trusting a well-intentioned person was not good enough when I arrived somewhere and couldn't get inside. Inevitably he or she would feel badly and so would I. It was irresponsible to put myself into impossible situations and expect other people to bail me out.

Unfortunately, the organized activities, though memorable, were not constant. Simply hanging out on a regular basis with fellow students was not a viable option in light of the fact that I lived at home. It was not possible to rearrange my paratransit ride or have one of my parents drive me at the drop of a hat. As a result, I wasn't exactly a fixture at informal get-togethers.

And it was too bad, because I made friends easily. While people always noticed my wheelchair, they quickly focused their attention elsewhere. One of my friends identified with me because we were both serious, highly-motivated students. Another was thrilled to meet a fellow journalism major and someone as passionate about sports as he was. Another friend and I enjoyed talking about our favorite hockey team, the Flyers, and whatever else was in the news. Friends and acquaintances knew me for much more than my wheelchair, even if I didn't realize it at the time.

The people I met in college accepted me much more easily than I had expected. Part of this had to do with the fact that in college, being different was celebrated. It was an atmosphere in which one could look at someone and think, "He sure is different, but that's okay. Good for him."

At Temple it seemed everyone I met had overcome something, whether it was an abusive situation, economic hardship, or racial, ethnic or sexual orientation difference. Disability was just one more item on the list. As one friend put it less than eloquently, "Everyone had problems, so it wasn't hard to fit in."

What I lost socially by not living on campus, I probably gained in terms of relationships with my family. I had the opportunity to spend a great deal of time with Mom, whose guidance and assistance proved invaluable. Now that I was an adult and had attendants to help me most of the time, she was more of a best friend than a caregiver.

I also had the chance to work on my relationship with Dad. Early in my college years, I remained resentful that he was not involved in my care. After an unrelated argument, we didn't speak to each other for nearly a week, which was possible because I really didn't need him for anything, or so I felt at the time.

In time my attitude changed. I realized that he was paying for my housing, education, and healthcare. More importantly, I still loved him. His comments and criticism over the years had driven me to succeed. I just needed to accept that there were certain things I could not change and that they were not worth sacrificing the entire relationship over.

I never did interact much with my sister Amy, who led a busy life in high school and had an active social life. I couldn't help but envy her, as she achieved milestones I had not, like learning to drive or going on a date.

On the other hand I had a chance to watch my youngest sister, Stephanie, grow up before my eyes. Many Saturday nights found the two of us ordering takeout food together. She helped me, albeit with some coaxing, get books or turn on my computer; I kept an eye on her. And whenever paratransit failed to show up, Mom had to drag her along. Trying to be a good big brother, I plied her with whatever gastronomic delights I could round up from the food carts at Temple.

I did regret being unable to get as involved socially as I would have liked when it came to girls. Even though I was good at making small talk and most of my college friends were girls, I was essentially shy and insecure, obsessing about what to say, how to say it, and when to say it. I spent class after class of a boring magazine writing course fantasizing about asking a cute classmate to get a cup of coffee with me. I spent so much time thinking about it that I never did ask her.

Occasionally, I overcame my fears and summoned the courage, like the time I asked a girl who escorted me on an elevator for a date. I kept thinking about asking, and finally did. She turned me down because she had a boyfriend, but told me that my wheelchair would not have been an issue.

Like she was going to actually say it was because I'm in a wheelchair. How stupid am I?

Though I did not spend much time thinking about sex, I did wonder about it and often read frank articles about sexuality in disability magazines, imagining the possibilities for me. Of course I always got bogged down in the details, like where we would get any privacy. Or if a girl's dorm room was accessible. Most importantly, how would I avoid injuring myself? After breaking my leg the way I had several years earlier, I didn't want to have to explain this one.

"Yeah, doc, my girlfriend was straddling me in my chair when we heard this cracking sound..."

But what I really wanted, what I longed for was the chance to be in a meaningful relationship where my needs were not the only issue. I didn't feel that any girl would be interested in me. Just as I wanted to be with an attractive girl, most girls had things they were looking for in a guy. I didn't think they were looking for a 110-pound guy with thin arms and legs, in a wheelchair and unable to take care of himself. That was just the kind of guy a girl wanted to bring home to meet her folks.

"So, son, what are your plans for the future?"

"Well, sir, I'll probably graduate and try to get a job. My health will get much worse and I'll be lucky to live another 10 years. Oh, and I live with my parents."

"Sounds great. My daughter is lucky to have met you."

And yet, I nearly had the kind of relationship I desired after meeting an outgoing, attractive girl in one of my classes. Leaving class together one day, we found we had a lot in common. A year younger than I, she had grown up in a nearby township and knew some people from my high school. We had similar social and political views, and were both studying communications at the time. She even knew a little bit about sports!

Eventually we talked on the phone a few days a week, engaging in fairly long conversations. I really enjoyed listening to what she said, and liked being able to offer advice and reassure her.

One thing we never discussed was my disability, although I often mentioned the attendant care problems I faced. I probably should have been more open about it, but my focus was on convincing people that I was not consumed with my disability. We didn't go out on any dates per se, though I once went to a basketball game with her. I was so self-conscious that I was afraid to ask for help getting food. Maybe it wasn't a date, but I didn't want it to look like I asked her just because I needed help. I could have asked one of the students who worked for me had that been the case.

I never tried to pursue a full-fledged relationship. Of course I had no idea whether she was even "interested" in me or if she simply liked me as a friend, which was more likely. I was afraid to ask, probably not unlike many guys. What made the situation worse was that I knew what the future had in store for me from a medical standpoint. I was not just a guy who happened to be in a wheelchair. This was someone I cared about, and she was going places. It was unreasonable to expect a girl like that to choose me over her goals. I would not have chosen me either had I been in her position. Still, I was afraid of having my heart broken over the reality of my disease.

Before long, my health situation prevented me from even trying. My occasional constipation problem worsened; I was tired and irritable and the last thing I wanted was to have a telephone conversation with someone, especially a girl I liked. Perhaps I should have explained what was happening, but I had never so much as mentioned my disease to her. And now I was going talk about my bowel issues? Who wanted to hear about that? It grossed me out! I could barely talk about it with doctors. I could only imagine the conversation.

"How was your day?" "Not great. I haven't gone to the bathroom for three days and my stomach is killing me, but thanks for asking."

Regardless of my social progress or lack thereof, my academic career was moving right along with most of my classes a part of my journalism major. Because the university was located in one of largest media markets in the country, Temple's journalism program was able to draw on professionals in the field and I had a chance to learn from newspaper editors and news broadcasters.

While I enjoyed most of my college classes, the practical nature of my journalism courses interested me the most. I was being prepared for a job in the field, and had every opportunity to learn what working in that field entailed. Whenever possible, professors assigned students to cover real-life stories.

Identifying myself as a freelance reporter rather than a student, I interviewed district attorneys, real estate developers, public advocates and baseball executives. Most interviews were conducted by telephone, which I loved because no one knew I was in a wheelchair. I was treated like any other reporter, for better or for worse.

I also learned to produce quality articles in a short period of time. I had always taken great pride in planning ahead so I wouldn't have to work on school assignments at the last minute. But in my journalism classes, there was no luxury of time between assignments. Surprisingly, it turned out that I worked well under pressure. I just *had* to complete assignments, but the perfectionist in me wouldn't allow myself to turn in anything less than my best.

I guess I had better get used to it. This is how it's going to be when I get out in the field.

That was when I realized I was not cut out for journalism. I could work under pressure, but it was not good for my health. When I was busy with my work, I did not take the time to eat or drink nor did I get enough sleep. It was a bad combination for anyone, let alone for someone with a serious disease.

As a journalist, I would not have had two other jobs and other classes, but I imagined that my assignments would be more involved and the deadlines even more immediate. I also thought about logistics. How was I going to get places when I had to cover events and interview people? Obviously everything couldn't be done by phone.

Fortunately I found another reason to abandon a career in journalism: my passion for the city. I had always been fascinated by the city of Philadelphia, particularly its history and future development. I wanted to understand why the economically depressed and drug infested North Philadelphia neighborhood surrounding Temple's campus was that way. I knew that my family had lived and worked there several decades earlier. As a journalism student, many of my assignments involved city issues such as waterfront development, the construction of sports stadiums, and the city's budding hospitality industry.

These were not merely assignments for me. I was legitimately interested in these issues and realized that I wanted to be more involved in them than merely writing about them. As a result, I began to seriously consider attending a graduate program in the study of city planning. I did not need to look very far, as I learned about the graduate program offered by Temple University's Department of Geography and Urban Studies. While not city planning, urban studies was a multi-disciplinary field that addressed employment, housing, and land-use among other issues which could lead to a career as an urban planner.

After meeting with the department chairman to get

a sense of the program, I knew it was the right fit for me and that it was convenient because my options were limited. Considering universities in other regions was not realistic. My health was not as good as it had been when I entered college, so I needed to be close to home. I didn't need the stress of finding help and adapting to a new place, nor did I want to look at other programs in the Philadelphia area. At Temple, everything was already familiar, particularly with regard to disability services.

Unlike the stress of choosing an undergraduate school, applying to graduate school was a simple process. I completed the application and was admitted several weeks later, relieved to have a sense of direction for the future. There was much less uncertainty than had I entered the job market. I could handle the academic world. That much I knew. The only question now was whether my health would cooperate.

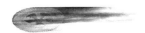

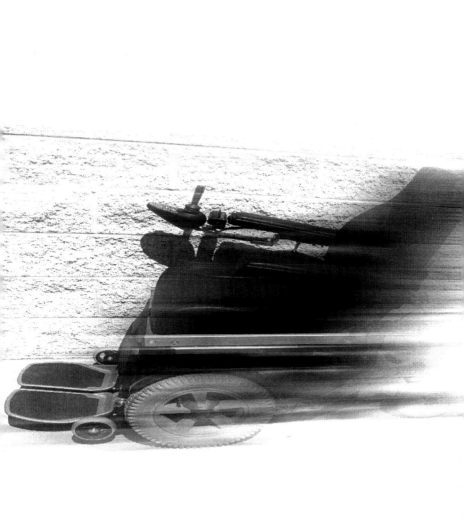

Going Downhill

10

The last thing I wanted to do when I was in college was focus on my health. I knew my disease would become more serious at some point, but that was years away. In the meantime, I would go as far as my body took me, pushing myself as hard as I could without worrying about the future.

There was no cure on the horizon, so I had no other choice but to get on with my life. Perhaps if I paid more attention to my work than to my health, I could somehow put off the serious aspects of my disease for a few more years.

When my health and education intersected, it was my education that won out. While on a bus trip to New York City, I hurt my lower back so badly that for the next two weeks driving my wheelchair over cracks in the sidewalk was torture. Riding to and from school in the back of a paratransit vehicle while Broad Street was being repaved was almost unbearable.

There was no choice except to grin and bear the pain. It was just before finals, I had assignments to complete, papers to write, and classes to attend.

Nobody wants to hear about it. I'll worry about it after finals, not now.

Unfortunately, it was impossible for me to concentrate. Not only was I in pain, but I was also consumed with fear that my spinal fusion might have somehow been damaged. What if surgery was necessary? The normal life I had built for myself would be destroyed and college would have to be put on hold. And go through that rehabilitation process again?

No way. I can't do that again. I won't do that again.

I hoped by ignoring the problem, it would go away. But it did not. Finally, I relented and went to see the orthopedist.

"That's the best job I ever did," the doctor remarked, as he reviewed the x-rays.

Glad you're impressed. Just tell me what the hell's wrong with my back.

Everything looked fine structurally, he told me. It was most likely a bad bruise that would heal in time. That was all I needed to hear. Miraculously my back began to feel better on the ride home, and by the following week things were back to normal. It felt as if I had dodged a bullet.

After that, I went back to avoiding the medical world

like the plague. When my neurologist took a position in another city, I stopped going to the muscular dystrophy clinic altogether.

Managing my cardiac and pulmonary issues was most important at this stage of the game, and I saw a pulmonologist at the hospital annually. Before I entered college, he assured my parents and me that any serious problems were five to six years away. As for my heart, I occasionally saw a cardiologist at the hospital and all indications were that I was doing as well as could be expected.

By the middle of my junior year, the stress of school, work and activities was beginning to catch up with me. I was so preoccupied that I didn't take the time to eat enough and began losing weight, more dramatically than I or Mom realized. We both bristled as Dad expressed concern when he saw my body as I was getting out of the shower one night. He was not involved in my day-to-day care, so what did he know? In reality, the fact that he did not see my body every day actually made him the best judge.

One of my advisors began noticing my weight loss as well. I had never really discussed my health with her and was uncomfortable doing so now. People already saw my wheelchair. The last thing I wanted was to appear any weaker. "I've probably lost a couple of pounds, but I'm okay," I said, minimizing her concern.

More than being too busy to eat, the occasional constipation problem that had bothered me for several years was growing more serious. Standard remedies like prune juice and stool softeners were no longer effective. I was often unable to fully relieve myself. The need to constantly go to the bathroom made eating uncomfortable. My stomach felt so full that I grew nauseated and was struggling to breathe. Ironically, I also experienced hunger pangs at the same time.

"I'm hungry; I don't think I had enough to eat," I complained to Mom.

"But you just said you were full," she said.

Calling the doctor about a fever or sore back was one thing. Talking about constipation was another story. I just couldn't bring myself to discuss it, preferring to have Mom do the talking.

The doctor prescribed a laxative that was so sickeningly sweet it made me gag if I didn't immediately chase it with a glass of water. Even then, I felt nauseated for the next hour or so. It seemed to help and that was all I needed to know. I also began eating cereal that was high in fiber and drinking cans of Ensure each day to supplement my diet. To chew the flakes I let them soften in milk, which made them absolutely gross. Between the medicine and the cereal, breakfast was truly delightful!

Although I didn't take the problem too seriously, my pulmonologist did. At my first visit with him a few years earlier, he had promised to focus not only on my pulmonary issues but on my overall health as well.

Now he followed through on his promise, demanding to know the reason I appeared to be losing so much weight.

"You hide it well," he said, pointing to the baggy long-sleeved shirt I was wearing on a warm day, "but come on, my three-year-old's arms are thicker than yours."

I hate the way my arms look. That's why they're covered. But do they look that bad?

"I've been having stomach problems so it's hard to eat a lot," I explained, too embarrassed to use the word "constipation."

I told him that the new laxative seemed to be helping and that I anticipated gaining weight.

"Alright, but this is something we need to watch," he warned.

His concern was that in an already compromised state, I would not have the "reserve" needed to fight off colds or more serious respiratory illnesses.

A few weeks later, I was still having the same problems. Tired of the almost constant abdominal discomfort and inability to eat, and afraid that something was seriously wrong we contacted the doctor, who ordered x-rays. We brought my Hoyer lift from home, and my parents somehow lowered me onto the cold, hard table even though the base of the lift didn't fit beneath the table. It was quite an ordeal, but I had put it off long enough.

After about an hour, the doctor huddled with us in the empty waiting room to discuss the results. While I did not have any serious problems, the x-rays revealed that my bowels were "filled with stool."

Isn't that special?

"We've known he's been full of it for a long time," Dad quipped, referring to what was in my head as opposed to my bowels.

I was not amused. Nor was I particularly excited by the doctor's plan, which went something like "take two enemas and call me in the morning."

Although that temporarily did the trick, my inability to fully relieve myself seemed to worsen after that. I should have bought stock in the Fleet enema company, as I used their product often over the next several months!

It was hardly a pleasant remedy. I was in the bathroom five or six times afterwards and the whole process took a tremendous toll on my body. My heart raced, I got light-headed and was so weak that I had to rest in bed for a few hours. It was also exhausting for Mom, who had to constantly wheel me in and out of the bathroom and then transfer me in and out of bed. Yet I was not especially concerned about my situation. I knew what the problem was and I was taking care of it.

But I was in the middle of my final semester and the pressure was starting to mount. With less energy to push myself than before, I made the decision to drop most of my classes, which was extremely disappointing. Two of the classes would have counted toward my American studies minor that now I would be unable to complete. But the second I dropped them, a weight was lifted from my shoulders and I could put my health before education.

In order to graduate however, I needed to complete a required newspaper layout course. The class itself was a piece of cake, but required every ounce of energy in me.

I used to be able to do so much. Now I can barely handle one class.

Classes were not the only thing I had to give up. With little energy to spare I stopped doing things I had taken for granted, like feeding myself. A few years earlier it would have been embarrassing to have someone else feed me, but now I needed to be practical. It simply required too much energy to bring a fork to my mouth, chew and swallow food. I did my best to ignore what this change represented, but this was a clear sign that my cherished independence was beginning to erode.

I also stopped writing, which didn't seem a big deal at the time. But soon I realized how much I missed being able to jot down a phone number or take notes when reading textbooks. The inability to type at the computer was of greater significance but thanks to modern technology, all hope was not lost.

After initially having my assistants type for me, I began using Dragon Naturally Speaking, a voice recognition program. With repeated usage, the program began to understand my voice and vocabulary. Dictating text rather than typing it took some adjustment. I was self-conscious of the fact that someone else could hear my thoughts at nearly the same time they entered my mind. Even with my bedroom door shut I was overly critical of myself, trying to be perfect when choosing my words.

I was able to get beyond that, but when confronted with the inaccuracy of the software I occasionally launched into expletive-laced tirades. And when it misinterpreted curse words, I grew enraged.

"Duck you, you stupid computer," it printed on the screen.

Damn it! All I want to do is curse at you and I can't even do that!

As spring arrived my health improved slightly, and before I knew it graduation day was upon me. I set aside my health concerns and embraced the moment. Proud of my academic achievements, I graduated summa cum laude with a perfect grade point average in my major. I was even prouder of how much I had grown, more confident, more assertive, and more independent than just a few years earlier. I had truly taken advantage of all the university setting offered.

The future looked bright, or so I thought, having no idea just how serious my health condition was. All of the evidence I needed could have been found in photos taken at my graduation party. I looked like a stick figure with a human head.

In spite of this, I couldn't have been any happier. I was surrounded by family, friends, professors and advisors and filled with a tremendous sense of accomplishment. I had gotten this far with few problems, and was convinced that I could complete graduate school and get a job before things got more serious. Little consideration was given to the fact that I was practically starving to death.

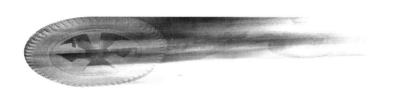

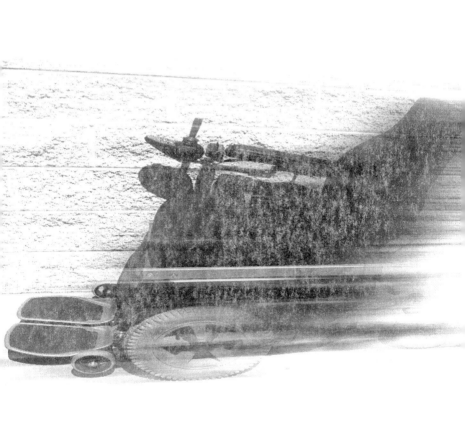

Student of the City

11

The chance to relax over the summer following college graduation seemed wonderful at first. No classes. No work. No stress. I could kick back and watch all of the baseball I wanted, even though the Phillies were awful that season. My bowel problems began to subside, as I took the time to eat properly and got used to the laxative medication.

But I was bored out of my mind! I had too much time to dwell on how I felt each day and focus on my shortcomings in life.

Though worried about not being able to push myself as I once had, I was ready to begin graduate school that fall. Besides, my internal clock was ticking, and I could not wait around until I felt perfect.

I'm still okay. I can finish my master's and get a job before things get serious.

Still, was this the right move? Was I going back to

school only because I was too afraid to try getting a real job? And urban studies? I was so tired of people asking, "What's that?" Or "What kind of a job can you get with that?" If I had any doubts, they quickly evaporated the moment I saw the department's course listings. I was like a kid in a candy store. There were classes on the ramifications of suburban sprawl, housing policy, economic development, and cities around the globe that I would never have the opportunity to visit. Once I actually started classes, there was no disappointment either.

Part of what made the program so appealing was its social conscience. Whatever the issue, consideration was given to its impact on impact on the poor, the elderly, immigrants, and minorities — groups often ignored by those with political or economic clout.

Many issues involved weighing the public interest against the interest of individual communities or residents. My disability made it easier for me to relate to those less fortunate. Though I led a life of privilege in many ways, I still knew what it felt like to be at a disadvantage in society.

I felt as little need as ever to prove myself to my classmates. It seemed obvious that everybody belonged, so I assumed they would apply that logic to me.

Successful in an academic environment for so long, I was beyond worrying about grades, confident that if I did my best work the grades would take care of themselves. Graduate school seemed to be a war of attrition anyway.

With challenging assignments to complete, the goal was to get things done.

That didn't mean that I didn't invest myself greatly into the issues raised. In assignments, I was dedicated to finding solutions to problems. My interests were far from academic. This was how I wanted to spend my life, however long it lasted, believing that working in this field would be a way of contributing to something greater than me. I did not want my life to always be about people helping me; I wanted to do something to make other lives better.

There were so many areas in which to make a difference: helping a community development group to revitalize a neighborhood, working on Philadelphia's campaign to recruit and retain young professionals, planning regional transportation, curbing suburban sprawl. Waterfront and park development intrigued me the most.

In nearly every city, waterfront areas were being reclaimed from industrial use for housing and recreation. Demand for parks, bicycle trails, and access to waterways was greater than ever. I envisioned helping to develop city parks and recreational areas where couples could embrace, parents could watch their children, and senior citizens could spend their golden years.

I would likely never fit into any of these categories, never have a girlfriend, never have kids, and never grow old and gray. But this was not about me. I didn't care if anyone ever knew my name. As long as people benefited from something I had done, that was all that mattered. The impact I could have on a city's landscape had the potential to last years after I took my last breath.

Although idealistic, I believed my dreams were realistic in the sense that I was not aiming to change the world, just a small part of it, and would have been content to stay at one position for many years as long as there continued to be new challenges. Because of my disease, I was better able to appreciate life's opportunities. While I would always work to achieve, the need to constantly look for something "better" was not paramount.

It was depressing that my health, particularly with its effect on my lifespan, was going to prevent me from achieving my goals.

This is just a pipe dream. Who am I kidding? I'm not going to have a chance to do these things.

Still, there were a couple of years before I needed to think about a career. In the meantime, I was busy enough with my daily routine as a graduate student. But even with the same drive and motivation I always had, my energy level was definitely not what it once was.

I was in a familiar setting, knew the process of hiring student workers to help me, was aware of the paratransit system, and thus was able to pick right up where I left off as an undergraduate student. It helped that I now traveled at off-peak hours being picked up at around 3 P.M., returning around 7:30 P.M. although paratransit wasn't any more reliable than it was in the past. There were times when I had to call Mom at nine o'clock, an hour and a half after my scheduled pickup time.

"Yeah, I'm still waiting here. They say the driver will be here soon."

"Do you want me to come down and pick you up?" she asked.

"No, no. I'm fine."

"It's already nine o'clock; you must be starving. I'll cancel your ride and pick you up."

"Well, if you insist..."

My class schedule was much different than it was in undergraduate school. Because my classes were late in the afternoon, I got up later and went to sleep later.

When I did have classes, I spent most of the day getting ready. My attendant got me dressed and in my wheelchair. I ate my fiber-laden breakfast and took my medicine, which made me get sick to my stomach and gag. I watched "SportsCenter" for an hour or so, trying to relax and conserve my energy. Sometimes, I tried to do some last-minute reading for class, but was too anxious to concentrate.

By early afternoon, my stomach was in knots, as I worried whether my paratransit ride was going to be on time. I choked down some lunch, even when I wasn't really hungry. If I didn't eat then, it would be several hours before I had the help or time to eat anything substantial. Mom helped me pack my books, put on my jacket, and attach my wheelchair tray.

After that, the waiting game began for my paratransit ride, which came on time if I was lucky. I rode to school already exhausted, and my day was just getting started.

One semester I had no choice but to schedule two classes back-to-back, each lasting two and a half hours. It would have been a lot for anyone. I didn't have a chance to eat beforehand and didn't dare drink more than a few sips of water because there was no time to go to the bathroom before class. By the end of the first class I was running on fumes, barely able to pay attention to the professor's words.

In order to have a break, I asked the professor to allow me to leave the first class early. One of my assistants met me, and we found someplace quiet to rest where he fed me a snack, usually something sugar-laden for an energy boost. It only made me feel nauseated, probably because I was in such a rush to get back to class.

I also used the bathroom, spending an inordinate amount of time in a stall with my assistant holding the urinal. I could only imagine how that looked when other people entered the restroom.

"Two guys in a stall. Get a room!"

If I did not go then, I had to wait another four hours (or five depending on paratransit) until I was home.

Think waterfalls! It's now or never. I am so late for class.

By the time I got home, I was in a daze and completely drained. While eating was generally a struggle for me, I had a voracious appetite on the days I had classes. I ate dinner in front of the TV with my parents, as we watched whichever local sports team was playing that night.

Exhausted each night as I got into bed, I had no regrets because my fatigue was a "good kind of tired."

I love what I'm doing. What's the alternative, anyway? Stay at home and rot?

Although school took a lot out of me, I felt that I needed to do more than just go to classes. Nearly every student I knew had some sort of job on campus. It seemed to be a normal part of graduate school life. I figured if they could handle it, so could I.

I had considered pursuing a graduate assistantship somewhere within the university, which would have paid my tuition. It also would have required a commitment of at least 20 hours a week.

While my head told me not to back away from such a challenge, my body convinced me that committing to something like that was insane. It would have been completely embarrassing to take a position and have to quit when it became clear that I had bitten off more than I could chew.

I ended up taking a job as a tutor at the university's writing center. What made the job unique was that my work was done online from home as part of the writing center's fledgling online tutoring service. Like the online courses I took as an undergraduate, working this way allowed me to be more productive by eliminating the hassle of commuting. The hours were very flexible; each semester I was assigned to work one or two days a week but never on days when I attended classes.

Though I enjoyed the work, it was more tiring than anticipated. While the rule of thumb was to spend no more than 45 minutes reviewing a student's paper and making comments, I needed to spend much longer because my voice recognition software was inaccurate. I spent an inordinate amount of time correcting its mistakes.

Even when the software was technically correct, it could be wrong. I told it to write, "Insert a comma here" and it wrote, "Insert a, here." As a result I tried to dictate less, opting instead to cut and paste whenever possible using the mouse, and at times cutting and pasting individual letters. It could be tedious, but there was no way I was going to make mistakes. I was supposed to be helping people fix their mistakes, not creating more!

Regretting not doing more from a social standpoint as an undergraduate, I felt far less pressure in graduate school. With classes and work, all I felt like doing in my spare time was watching sports and sleeping. The bottom line was that it was enough that I loved what I was doing with my life. I was going to be the type of person whose life would be focused on his career, anyway. I was never going to be a social animal.

It was not as if I was missing out on much. Some of my classmates were already professionals in the field with busy schedules and families; they were not in school for a social experience. The other full-time students were also busy with internships and jobs.

Similar to my undergraduate years, I became so obsessed with school that my health became secondary. It was over the summer between my first and second years of graduate school that I began to at least consider my health issues a bit more.

Though my bowel problems of the previous year had diminished, I was still vastly underweight. At the urging of my pulmonologist, I agreed to meet with a nutritionist. Because the muscles I used for breathing were growing weaker, the nutritionist explained that I was expending calories just to breathe, which was why I was having such a hard time gaining weight.

My caloric requirements were therefore higher, although she stressed the need to increase my intake slowly in order to avoid a potentially fatal complication known as "re-feeding syndrome" in which taking in too much too quickly resulted in significant electrolyte imbalance and dangerous irregular heart rhythms, among other problems.

The trick was simply finding versions of foods I already ate that were higher in calories and fat. The nutritionist recommended using whole milk with cereal and switching from margarine to butter. Ordinarily, this would have horrified Mom, whose recipes came from Weight Watchers cookbooks.

"Can you eat foods with more salt, more fat? Do you ever eat fast food?" she asked me after consulting with my cardiologist.

Lady, are you kidding? I'm a college student!

It was the kind of diet most people would kill for. My biggest concern every night was which gourmet ice cream I should eat: Godiva, Ben & Jerry's, or Haagen-Dazs. If I wanted eggs for breakfast that was what I ate, prepared with milk and butter of course. If Mom prepared a meal served over brown rice, I ate a saltier, higher calorie flavored rice instead, and when the mood struck me for a late-night slice of pizza, I never hesitated.

I looked for extra calories wherever I could, whether it meant washing my food down with fruit juices instead of water or opting for the creamier New England clam chowder instead of chicken noodle soup when deciding what to have for lunch.

In my holiday newsletter that year, I joked, "I know, I know. It's really difficult eating fried chicken and gourmet ice cream all the time, but I'm trying..."

The truth of the matter was that it *was* difficult. I could only eat tiny portions and at times began to feel uncomfortable after only a few bites. I struggled to finish a piece of chicken. Already full from dinner, I hardly considered ice cream a treat.

My nutritionist and pulmonologist both suggested admitting me to the hospital for a week or so for what they termed a "nutritional evaluation." My condition would be monitored as my caloric intake was increased. A feeding tube was discussed, but it was not emphasized. Basically, the plan sounded like more of the same thing I was already doing at home.

"I'm not trying to be difficult. It's just that if I can't gain weight eating things I like at home, I'm probably not going to do any better eating hospital food," I reasoned.

More than that, I did not want what seemed a relatively minor issue to interfere with my life, and was far more concerned with the statistics class I was taking that summer. Surely my health was not great, but I was still going to live on my own terms. Spending time in the hospital was not part of the plan.

By making my health a higher priority, I would cease to have a normal outlook on life, spending my days obsessed with how I was feeling rather than actually accomplishing anything.

Maybe it would be better to go all out. Use every bit of energy — even if it kills me.

While I did not agree with the nutritionist to be admitted to the hospital, I promised to make a concerted effort to work on my nutrition.

I did agree to an overnight stay at the hospital for a sleep study. My pulmonologist had lobbied me hard for the study, in which my breathing would be monitored while I slept. The study's findings would be used to determine if I needed any sort of equipment to assist in my breathing at night.

I had no idea how impossible it would be to actually sleep during a sleep study. In the first place, the study began much earlier than the time I usually fell asleep. When I tried to fall asleep, the conditions were unbearable. The room was too cold, the bed was uncomfortable, and the pillows were too firm. Worse, my body was covered with annoying probes and wires. How could anyone sleep for even five minutes?

Sleep study, my ass!

Sometime around 6 A.M., the time I typically fell into

a deep sleep, the technician woke me up. "Okay, we're finished here," he announced.

What? But I just fell asleep. Don't you want to monitor me while I'm actually asleep?

Not surprisingly, the test indicated that I had slept only half the time. There were some minor abnormalities, but nothing that my doctor felt needed assistance from a machine. Though glad about the doctor's conclusion, I had my doubts as to the accuracy of the study, having never had the chance to settle into a deep sleep.

———————•———————

During my second year in graduate school it was time to get serious about a thesis topic. Initially I decided that I wanted to focus on the economic impact of urban universities on their surrounding communities.

Though it was an interesting topic, I realized it would be very difficult physically. It was not the kind of research I could do from a telephone. The kinds of places I would have to visit were not going to be wheelchair accessible. I hated to let my disability prevent me from doing something, but needed to be realistic.

In keeping with the city-university relationship, or "town-gown" as it was often called, I decided to investigate whether universities used their location in or near cities to attract students and if so, how? I considered university websites, as the Internet was the medium of choice for most young people.

It was a perfect project for me in that I would never need to leave home to visit websites. With my advisor's blessing, I began researching background material and planned to conduct my study over the summer.

During winter break, I had an encouraging visit with my pulmonologist. My new diet had apparently been working to the tune of nine pounds gained in six months. This pleased the doctor, who chuckled at the sight of Mom feeding me a sandwich in the middle of my appointment.

"Sorry," I explained between bites, "I was too hungry to wait."

"Whatever you're doing, it's working. Keep it up," he encouraged me.

I beamed with pride. I was in the planning stages of my thesis with an anticipated completion by the summer, and fall graduation. Then I would evaluate my situation before moving forward with my life.

Unfortunately, my body proved unwilling to cooperate. Before I knew it, everything got worse. The constipation that I had been able to control stopped responding to the medication, and it became more difficult than ever to eat. My pulmonologist switched me to a stronger laxative. It had some effect, but by then it was probably too late to stop me from losing weight.

My respiratory status started to take a nose dive. One of the clearest signs was that for the first time, I began having trouble projecting my voice, most notably when riding in paratransit vehicles. Having conversations with drivers over the sound of the engine was exhausting. I frequently felt short of breath, often feeling heart palpitations. I went to bed exhausted but struggled to fall asleep, partly out of fear of not waking up the next day. Eventually, I fell asleep anyway.

To hell with this. I don't care if I don't wake up. I'm too tired. I'm going to sleep.

Most mornings I woke up with a headache. Many mornings I woke up with phlegm in my chest. If it stayed there, I risked developing pneumonia. Even with a weak cough, I forced myself to cough for hours on end until my chest was clear and I had swallowed much of it.

Well, I'm certainly not hungry now!

I could barely handle the one class in my schedule that semester. On the way home I was so exhausted that I became entranced by the traffic lights, wanting to simply collapse. Fortunately, it was the last class necessary for my graduate program. After that, I would be able to work exclusively on my thesis.

I figured that without the stress of commuting to campus, I would still be well enough to finish my thesis by the end of the summer. I was wrong.

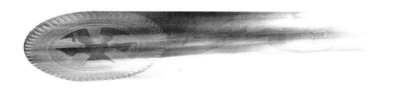

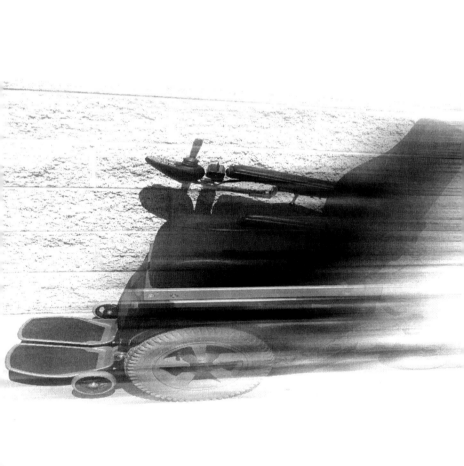

The Visit

12

"Deep breath in! Now push... push... push... push... push!" the respiratory therapist coached me, as I completed another round of pulmonary function testing.

Breathless and exhausted, I looked up at the computer screen to see how I had done, but couldn't understand what anything meant.

"Good job," he said as he printed the test results for my pulmonologist.

But he was just being kind. In the past, I had often worried that my performance on the tests would not accurately reflect my condition. I typically did worse when it was extremely humid or cold outside or when I had stayed up late the night before. Considering how short of breath and lethargic I had been feeling lately, the results were definitely on target this time.

Even more alarming than the test results was my

weight. According to the clinic's scale, I had lost almost all of the weight gained since my previous visit a few months earlier. I weighed a ghastly 69 pounds.

All that hard work down the drain.

I hung my head as I waited with my parents to see the doctor. There was no escaping the fact that I was in bad shape.

When the nurse practitioner visited with us a few minutes later, she went through the usual questions about my breathing, my sleeping patterns, my appetite, and my general level of energy. Though not particularly cheerful, I tried to be as forthcoming as possible.

Based on what I told her, she mentioned the possibility of some form of a non-invasive ventilation device, a breathing machine with a mask to help me rest better at night so I would have more energy during the day. Some of my friends with Duchenne had been using such devices for several years.

When the nurse practitioner left the room to consult with the doctor, I was relieved that some new equipment might be all that was needed. But would it make a difference? I had been feeling so awful lately. It had been a struggle to physically get through one class this semester. Was this equipment really going to be enough?

Oh, come on. Do I really want something more? Maybe I'm making too big of a deal about this...

At that moment the door swung open and the doctor entered the room, the nurse practitioner and the pulmonary clinic social worker behind him. He wasted no time.

"Joshua, I've always been honest with you because you're not a child," he said in his distinctive Israeli accent. "It isn't easy for me to say this because I know you have tried hard. And I have tried to wait as long as possible, but now is not the time to wait anymore."

My respiratory and nutritional status was at a critical point and required a major intervention. I needed a tracheostomy and use of a ventilator at least part of the time. For a few hours of the day, I would likely be able to come off the machine and breathe on my own or "sprint."

To address my poor nutrition, I also needed a feeding tube placed directly into the stomach (commonly known as a "g-tube"), which would allow me to receive much more nutrition than eating by mouth.

If I waited even a few months, I would be unlikely to live for more than a very short time. By acting now, I could live another five, six, or more years with a relatively good quality of life, according to the doctor.

It was a shock to hear my life expectancy discussed. Although I was certainly aware of the reality, no doctor had ever discussed it with me before. Of course, I had been doing well for so long that it had not been much of an issue. For the first time in my life, my disease had become life-threatening.

Wow. We've reached that point.

"It's not a perfect solution," said the doctor, "but it's the best that modern medicine has to offer, and I strongly recommend that we take advantage of it."

My parents, sitting to my right, listened with concern but said nothing. I dared not look at them for more than a second, fearing I would get choked up. I needed to be strong for them and to remind myself that I was a mature adult who could handle bad news.

But as I tried to speak, tears began to well up in my eyes. All I could do was nod in agreement, telling the doctor, "I agree... I agree."

After a few seconds, I was able to venture a bit further. "I've actually heard some people say that [a tracheostomy] was the best thing to happen to them, that they were able to become *more* independent."

Whether this was directed at the doctor or my parents, I was trying to think of something positive to say. Otherwise, I might have been completely overcome by my emotions.

At the same time, I felt validated. Something was seriously wrong with me and there was no way around it. Moreover, I felt a tremendous sense of relief. I had been preparing for this moment for some time, and knew I would eventually need these procedures and would agree to them when the time came. Now that time had arrived. The black cloud hanging over my head had been lifted and I would be able to get used to the way the rest of my life was going to be.

The conversation then shifted to the planning phase. I would need to prepare for a hospital stay of perhaps as long as two months. The surgery itself would be quick, after which I would spend several days recovering in the intensive care unit. I would then be transferred to a rehabilitative unit in the adjacent Children's Seashore House, where my parents would become trained in my care and during which time my home nursing care would be arranged.

Eligible for 16 hours of nursing care a day which would be vital, I would no longer be able to stay by myself or with anyone not trained in my care. Someone would also need to stay awake at night while I slept, mostly in case my ventilator malfunctioned.

The social worker warned us that arranging nursing care would be what kept me in the hospital for so long, in light of the fact that there was a severe nursing shortage.

When I asked how soon surgery would be, the doctor told me that the situation was "urgent, but not an emergency." Everything could be arranged by the end of the month. Still, he advised me against taking a trip that I had planned to Boston to see some baseball and visit with friends the following week.

"There will be plenty of time for baseball games later," he said.

Yeah, sure.

A six hour trip was difficult enough for me now. How was I going to travel on a ventilator? I was disappointed, but it wasn't the end of the world. I certainly did not want to be out of town if my condition suddenly took a turn for the worse.

Before he left the room, I asked the doctor if the two procedures were reversible; he assured me that they were. Though I had no reasonable expectation of living to see a cure that would make these interventions no longer necessary, I wanted to keep my options open regardless of how slim the chances.

I also asked if I would be able to talk or eat with the trach. Being unable to speak would completely change my personality; and while eating had not been easy in recent years, it hadn't been for lack of desire.

While there was no absolute guarantee, the doctor told me I would be able to do both. However, I would probably be unable to speak for at least the first couple of days after surgery due to swelling.

That night, Mom began calling various family members as well as some of the other Duchenne families we knew who had already been through what we were about to experience. I tried to relax in front of the TV, tuning into the NBA Finals featuring the New Jersey Nets versus the Los Angeles Lakers. How different from last year when my hometown 76ers had been in the finals and things were so much better for me. I had just completed my first year of graduate school and was hopeful about my future. My health was not great, but I was beginning to gain weight and thought I'd be able to complete my master's degree before having to worry about anything serious. The world itself was so different then; the September 11th attacks had not yet occurred.

Over the next few weeks, my condition continued its steady decline and I began to wonder if it was safe for me to remain at home. Mom and I concluded that the doctor would not have let me leave the hospital after my checkup if he thought that my life was in danger. I sure hoped he was right.

No measurements were recorded, but I knew that I was still losing weight. Trying to eat was an exercise in futility, even more difficult than during earlier times when I had lost weight. The less I ate, the less of an appetite; when I was actually hungry, the abdominal discomfort felt after eating a small amount of food forced me to stop. And still, I felt hunger pangs.

The shortness of breath I had occasionally experienced over the past few years was now a major problem. Often too tired to dictate to the computer or have conversations with people, I went to bed exhausted and woke up feeling virtually the same. Sleep, when it came, was not restful, but the dead-tired kind of sleep that is necessary when catching up. More alarmingly, my heart raced almost constantly, no doubt due to the fact that my body's electrolytes were out sync from lack of nourishment. The only thing that seemed to help was drinking glass after glass of Gatorade.

The obvious decline in my health over only a couple weeks since my pulmonary clinic visit made it vital that my admission to the hospital take place sooner rather than later. Dad called the doctor's office, stressing that I had basically stopped eating and they agreed to admit me a week earlier.

While my physical decline during this period of time was dramatic, the emotions I felt were equally compelling. I had worked hard to establish my lifestyle, while keeping my disease out of it as much as possible. Now, my disease was threatening to destroy me if I did not confront it. I was going to have to put my life on hold, with the realization that even afterwards it would never be the same. As much as I had anticipated that this time would come, now that it was here I wasn't sure I was ready for it.

Never before had my disease made me feel like a sick person. People with other diseases were "sick." Whenever I had started to feel sorry for myself before, I realized how fortunate I was in so many ways. My disease was a life-threatening condition, but until now death had seemed light years away. Now I was seriously ill. I was getting a trach, something reserved for a serious situation. What had seemed so far away had been reduced to five or six years. It was all so unsettling.

Regardless of how much time I had left, I was going to make the most of it. For now, though, I busied myself preparing for my "summer vacation." I did not have a full-time job, a family to feed, or a mortgage to pay, but I still had obligations that required my attention.

I contacted my graduate advisor to inquire about taking a leave of absence from my studies. Though I had never shared much about my disease with my professors, my e-mail explained that what I was about to go through was not uncommon for someone with my disease and that I had every intention of returning to complete my degree.

Shortly thereafter, I received an encouraging response

from the professor, stressing that I was a "valued member of the department" and that they would do whatever it took to keep me.

I also informed the director of the university writing center that I would be leaving my tutoring job. I had no idea how much I was going to miss the feeling of self-worth that came from being employed.

One of the most important things I did was craft an e-mail to as many friends, family members, and professors as possible. I didn't want to discuss too much about my disease; it wasn't something on which I wanted to dwell. I had never done so in the past and was not about to start now.

At the same time, I needed to provide information to people who cared about me and who would want to know what I was now facing. I had little energy to dictate my message to the computer, but did not want people to find out from someone else and therefore pushed myself just as I had done many times before.

The many heartfelt responses received made me glad I had chosen to communicate frankly with others about my situation rather than hiding it from the people who cared about me. I was going to need all the support I could get and people would be unable to help unless they knew I needed it.

One of the most helpful messages came from my friend Brian, who already had a tracheostomy and a feeding tube. Whenever I had needed advice about my disease in the past, I had always turned to Brian and his brother, Michael. After Mom contacted their mom, Brian wrote to me.

Dear Josh,

I know this must be a hard time for you and your family. I remember how hard it was to breathe before my surgery. I also lost 40 pounds in a short time when I was having trouble breathing. When I had my surgery done I was out of work for a short time, and was able to return without any problems.

Michael and I would be glad to meet with you and your family either at my house or yours. Let me know when you want to do this, my house would be better so you will be able to see our home and travel equipment.

~Brian

Reading Brian's message made the upcoming ordeal seem much more bearable. How bad could any of this really be if Brian had such positive things to say?

On an extremely hot and humid afternoon, my parents and I visited with Brian, his brother, and their parents at their home. Due to the weather conditions, I struggled mightily to breathe, but noticed that my friends seemed to have no trouble at all, thanks to their ventilators. I could not wait to be able to breathe that easily. We saw how small their ventilators were, able to fit on the back of their wheelchairs.

The machines were not necessarily quiet, especially with two of them running at the same time. Their mom joked that if the TV was on and her sons entered the room, she would have to raise the volume in order to hear. We saw the brothers' bedrooms, with ventilators next to their beds and suction machines and emergency supplies nearby. None of the equipment took up much space.

There was a large cabinet in which medical supplies such as dressings, tracheostomy tubes, and additional tubing for the ventilators were stored. My friends' mom removed a trach from the supply cabinet to show me what it looked like. Sealed in its sterile packaging, the curved tube was no more than a few inches long.

"It's much smaller than you probably thought. I was surprised about that myself," she said.

She was right. I had envisioned a much longer tube that would extend far into my trachea or windpipe. I also had not realized that the tube would need to be changed on a regular basis. That didn't sound like a whole lot of fun, but if that was part of living with a trach then I would just have to get used to it.

How bad could it really be?

I asked the brothers about the surgery itself. They told me it was not especially painful, although they warned that the area in my abdomen around the feeding tube would initially be very sore. I hoped they were right about it not being too painful.

Dad spent some time talking with my friends' dad, who suggested that we purchase a gas-powered generator in the event of a prolonged power outage. I had not thought of how I would power my ventilator once its batteries were depleted. He told us about the first snowstorm that they needed to run the generator. "We were the only people on the block who could watch TV," he told us with a proud smile.

Our visit to my friends' home offered helpful information and reassurance that things were not as bleak as they seemed. I felt much better afterward and sensed that Mom, initially overwhelmed by the thought of so much to learn, also felt better.

I was about to begin a new chapter in my life, another step on my journey. There was no turning back.

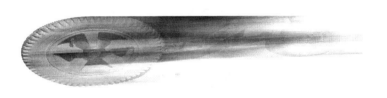

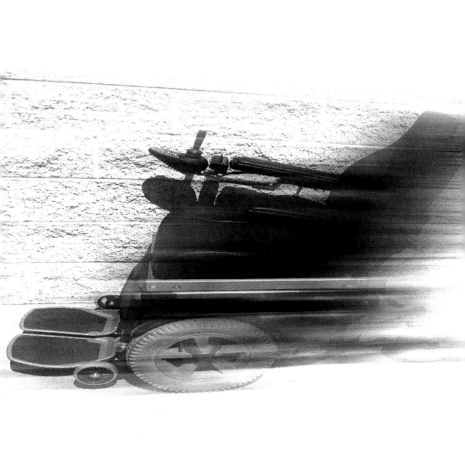

Man on a Mission

13

By the time I was admitted to the hospital I had hardly eaten for days, surviving on chicken noodle soup, applesauce, yogurt, and Gatorade by the bottle. I had nearly thrown up that morning after only a few mouthfuls of soup, and felt my heart beating in my throat. Without medical attention, I knew it was only a matter of time before something serious would happen to me.

Arriving at the hospital, the hot, suffocating air hit me the second I got out of the van. It was definitely summertime in Philadelphia. I looked up at the red brick building, never so glad to be at a medical facility. Waiting for my parents to unload my bags, each breath I took was more difficult than the one before. I was so hungry I wanted to pass out. There was no time to be scared or depressed. I was on a mission to save my life. Somehow

I would get nutrition into my body. I was at the hospital, and it would be their problem now.

Perhaps I should have paused for a moment to reflect on what I was about to lose, but I thought I could handle anything. I had no regrets about the surgery; if I wanted to live, it had to be done. I didn't take the time to consider that my self-image, independence, and lifestyle were never going to be the same.

The only thing on my mind was that I was starving. By the time we reached the admissions office, my patience was already wearing thin. I didn't care what I signed, even if it meant selling my soul to the devil; I was going to get something to eat!

Although it seemed to take forever, all of the required paperwork was eventually completed and I was admitted to the hospital. I saw many people that day, but couldn't wait to see the nutritionist. I told her how hungry I was but doubted that I could take much by mouth, as chewing and swallowing had become nearly impossible.

She explained that while I was waiting for the surgery to place a feeding tube in my stomach, I could have a tube inserted through my nose, down my throat and esophagus, and into my stomach. It didn't sound like fun, but desperate times called for desperate measures so I agreed to it.

As I lay in a reclined position, a cute young nurse leaned over me and began inserting the thin, well-lubricated tube up my nose.

"Okay. Now...swallow...swallow...swallow," she coached me.

It felt like a strand of spaghetti in the back of my throat that wouldn't go down. I gagged, but it wasn't really so bad. Plus, there was a cute nurse hovering over me, and that could never be bad! The tube was taped in place and connected to a feeding pump. Within an hour, my hunger pangs began to subside as an off-white colored liquid filled with much-needed nutrients slowly dripped into my stomach. It felt cold and was basically tasteless, but I could detect a slight vanilla taste if I concentrated hard enough. I began to relax. My heart stopped racing and I started feeling more energetic.

Though exhausted from the day's events, I couldn't fall asleep that night. This didn't exactly surprise me, as I often had trouble falling asleep in my own bed. Against my better sense, I allowed the doctor to talk me into taking some medication to help me sleep. I had never liked taking medications, no matter how safe they were considered. I was given Benadryl, which typically causes drowsiness, apparently except in me.

After initially falling into a deep sleep, I suddenly woke up a raving lunatic, animatedly asking Mom all sorts of crazy questions.

"Where am I? Why am I here?" I demanded to know. There was no reasoning with me.

"But I don't understand," I persisted, "Why am I here?"

I grew increasingly agitated before finally giving up and drifting back to sleep. Nurses and doctors were called and it was determined that the medicine had caused a "paradoxical reaction." Instead of helping me sleep, it had done the exact opposite, making me completely nuts.

Though ready to do whatever was necessary to get on with my life, beneath the surface I was more anxious than I realized. I might have been unable to articulate my fears, but my brain was not about to stay silent.

The next couple days preparing for surgery were far worse than the surgery itself. Preoperative tests considered "routine" by doctors, nurses, and technicians were anything but. There were few explanations as to the purpose of the tests. Some of them were uncomfortable, and some of the people performing them seemed to think that I was being difficult when I complained of discomfort. As if they would have handled it any better.

The upper GI study, which allowed doctors to check the position of my stomach, turned out to be a major ordeal. First, I had to ingest a solution containing barium, a contrast agent that would stand out in an x-ray.

The real fun began when it was time to transfer me from my wheelchair to the x-ray table. As I looked at the table, I knew there was no way my Hoyer lift was going to reach the table. There was no way I was going to let anyone lift me onto the table out of fear that my knees would be accidentally stretched too far.

Somehow, Mom and my aunt who had come to visit positioned the lift around the corner of the table, raised me as far as possible and slid me onto the table as the chains from the lift threatened to strangle us all. Meanwhile, the nurses and technicians tried to help them position me using pillows and blankets. I was a nervous wreck, driving everyone crazy.

"Watch my legs... watch my legs... watch my legs!" I hollered.

Once on the table, my hips and legs could not rest properly and my back was killing me. The only way to get any relief was to keep my legs elevated.

The doctor entered the room and matter-of-factly told me to roll onto my right side. As if I could even do that myself.

"But I can't roll that way," I explained.

He was less than pleased. "Then we can't do the test," he said, as the right side was the direction in which the stomach emptied. There had to be some other way. I hadn't been able to lay on my right side in years. Finally, the doctor allowed me to simply elevate my upper body on a slight angle using pillows.

"This could take hours," he muttered, "and we don't have that kind of time. There are others waiting."

You know what? I don't care about them right now.

As it turned out, even in this position it barely took 20 minutes for the barium to move as required, probably because my stomach was so small from malnourishment.

Well, what do you have to say for yourself now?

Getting off of the table was nearly as difficult as getting on. Before leaving the room, I asked a nurse if the barium had any side effects.

"Not really," she said, "although it could cause some constipation."

Great. I've never had that problem before.

Actually, going to the bathroom was not a problem that night although I did not feel completely relieved. I didn't give it another thought, nor did anyone else. I would pay for that.

When I returned from the test, a doctor pulled us aside. When we told him about the ordeal we had just endured, he seemed to feel badly.

"It didn't absolutely have to be done if it was that much trouble," he said.

That would have been nice to know about three hours ago!

According to the doctor, it was apparently not going to be possible for me to have surgery the following day due to a shortage of available operating rooms. It was not necessarily the worst thing for me anyway, he explained. This way, I could continue to receive nutrition and build up my strength for the surgery. He said he could write a note allowing me to come and go from the hospital.

It sounded reasonable enough. I wanted to get everything over with as soon as possible, but maybe it would be a good idea to wait.

And just as soon as I had reconciled this turn of events, another doctor came and turned my world upside down. "We can do your surgery tomorrow if you still want," he said.

"But the other doctor said it might be better to wait," I explained.

"Never mind with that; we can do it *tomorrow,*" the doctor snapped. "Well... uh... uh..." I stammered. "Come on," he interrupted. "You need to make a decision now. If you're not ready, we're going to have to give the space to somebody else."

Backed into a corner, I angrily replied, "Okay, *fine* I'll do it." I was fuming. There was no doubt in my mind that I was going to say yes. All I wanted was 30 seconds before I agreed to sign away my life, no matter how small the risks.

It's my body, not yours. And don't talk to me about other people. I can't be a little bit selfish at a time like this?

As I drove my wheelchair back to my room to settle in for the evening, I realized that the first doctor had simply been trying to lessen my disappointment at a possible delay in surgery. I didn't actually need to build up my strength for the operation. He had not been completely honest with me, and I was glad. I couldn't have handled the truth at that moment.

Although it took some time, I eventually fell asleep that night without any drugs, thank you very much. Sometime in the early morning hours, two pretty female doctors entered my room. I had been asleep, but they had my immediate attention. After all, I had been asleep, not dead!

It turned out that they were not there for my good looks or my charming personality. They needed to draw some blood to avoid any delay in my surgery in the morning. And there was no phlebotomist available for the task, which I later learned was not exactly true. I knew that phlebotomists and nurses were typically better than doctors when it came to drawing blood, but said nothing.

By the third or fourth try Mom, now awakened, had grown impatient with them and insisted that they find a nurse. I was much more patient and allowed them to continue. If they had been fat and ugly, I would have given them a much shorter leash!

The next morning, an old family acquaintance who was an anesthesiologist at the hospital greeted me and my parents in the preoperative area and said that he would take me back. I asked him about his son who had graduated high school the year before I had, and he told me that he was getting married soon. I couldn't help but feel a bit sad. His son and I were basically the same age, but we were miles apart in terms of our lives. I wished I was the one getting married and looking forward to a promising future.

I repeated a request already made several times, to be "knocked out" before being transferred to the operating table. I was terribly afraid of being moved without my Hoyer lift.

Then, it was time to go. I didn't feel particularly emotional. Obviously there were risks with any surgery, but they were relatively small. I had every reasonable expectation that I would wake up. Mom planted a kiss on my forehead and the doctor began wheeling me down the hallway.

Once inside the operating room, a number of nurses and doctors were there to greet me. Unlike ten years earlier when I had back surgery, I had little interest in the anesthesia process. All I wanted was to get on with the surgery and with feeling better.

I glanced at the operating table to my left, glad that I would be asleep when they transferred me. If I was hurt I wouldn't feel a thing, at least not until later.

The next thing I knew, I woke up gasping for breath. "I can't breathe!" I tried to say, but couldn't talk. Actually I was breathing with the help of a nurse "bagging" me with a rubber device that was operated by hand, squeezing air into my lungs intermittently. It was uncomfortable, and I was glad to fall back asleep.

It was dramatically better the next time I awoke. My parents were at my bedside, and I was able to talk with no problem at all! My voice was even stronger than prior to the surgery. I was so relieved to be able to speak. How awful it would have been if I couldn't communicate with doctors, nurses, and others involved in my care during recovery.

Resting in bed, I felt so comfortable breathing. Mom saw an immediate difference, noting that the coloring had returned to my face. Though the ventilator sounded much like the turbine of an airplane, the white noise it created was actually rather calming. All I wanted to do was talk, so much so that when my pulmonologist visited, he basically told me to shut up. "You need to rest," he said. "There will be plenty of time to talk later."

I was in far less pain than I remembered from my spinal fusion. My trach site hardly hurt at all, which was rather surprising to me. I would have thought that a hole in my neck would be highly painful. There was some pain where my g-tube had been inserted, just as my friends had warned, but all I needed was some Tylenol, although it had to be given rectally since I couldn't swallow and my g-tube wasn't ready for use. Hardly pleasant, but neither was being in pain, so it was a necessary evil.

That night, I received my introduction to the wonderful world of suctioning. Because the trach was a foreign material in my body, the body produced extra secretions, or mucus. When the secretions built up in the trach, it became harder to breathe. Sometimes I could cough the secretions into my mouth and swallow them, but my cough was usually too weak to do so. So the nurse inserted a thin plastic catheter connected to a suction machine, which pulled the secretions out of my trach. It caused me to cough and my tongue to stick out involuntarily. My eyes watered and I gagged. It was a bit uncomfortable, but when the trach was "junky," I felt much better after suctioning.

In time, I would require little in the way of suctioning (only a few times a day as opposed to people who needed it several times *an hour*). But since I was just getting used to the trach, my body produced a great deal of secretions in the first week after surgery, so much that I needed to have my nose and throat suctioned as well.

If all went according to plan, I would spend a few days in intensive care, and after a successful first trach change be moved to the hospital's rehabilitative unit. There, my family would be trained in my care and I would stay until home nursing care could be arranged.

But in the hospital things don't always go according to plan, as I would soon find out.

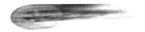

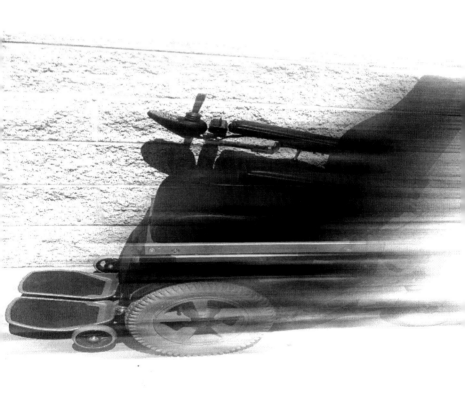

14

It was time to eat. Following about a day in which my g-tube was not yet allowed to be used, I was cleared to begin "feedings."

Great. That doesn't make me seem like a baby — feedings.

It was assumed that I would be able to handle about three ounces per hour at the very least. At first, I tolerated it well, but soon began to feel extremely bloated and uncomfortable. Initially, doctors chalked my discomfort up to the fact that I was not used to having so much in my tiny stomach and needed time to adjust.

Sounded like a logical explanation. I had no reason to doubt it, as everything was new to me. When I continued to complain of discomfort however, another explanation was identified, excess gas caused by the "formula." To resolve this issue, a port in the feeding tube was connected to an open syringe that hung from an IV pole. It didn't help all that much. Another thought was that my discomfort was due to the fact that my bladder was full. I had not been able to pee for several hours.

"We could cath you," said the hulking *male* nurse.

"Well, if you think it might help, I guess," I said, more concerned that a guy was going to violate me than about the general unpleasantness of being catheterized.

When it was repeated several hours later by a pretty female nurse, I was only wishing for a male nurse or at least an ugly female one. I was getting aroused as she inserted the catheter and pushed gently on my stomach with her hand. Not only was it embarrassing, it was making the insertion process a lot more uncomfortable.

I'm not interested. I'm not interested. I'm not interested.

I tried to relax, but couldn't help it. I was a 24-year-old heterosexual male. If only I was somewhere else and my "excitement" was for another, much better reason.

Still, the abdominal discomfort persisted. The doctors and nurses were starting not to believe me. Sure, they were used to taking care of children, but I was no child. There was no way I was exaggerating and my patience was starting to wear thin.

Finally, x-rays were ordered. Sure enough, something was up. It was the revenge of the barium! The solution given to me a couple of days earlier during my upper GI study had not been completely cleared out of my system. Then I had surgery and the anesthesia had slowed everything down, and I had not moved my bowels since. The resident handling my case explained that barium, if it stayed in one's system for some time, hardened much like concrete and could make it difficult for waste to pass around it. That was why I was feeling such discomfort.

I was given a vast array of laxatives, seemingly from every imaginable orifice. Everything short of dynamite (my suggestion) was tried with little or no effect. I tried to laugh about it, but I was feeling anything but funny. Eventually, it was the old standby Fleet enema that seemed to do the trick (sounds like an endorsement). It was a good thing, too because when I asked him what the next weapon in the arsenal was, the young doctor said they could give me a milk and molasses enema.

"You're kidding," Dad and I said in unison.

"Seriously, it works," he said.

How delicious!

I wasn't allowed to get out of bed and couldn't sit on a bedpan because it rubbed against my back, causing excruciating pain. So I was turned on my side. Diapers and towels were slid underneath me, and well you can figure out the rest. Gross as it was, I finally felt some relief. Unfortunately, a repeat x-ray several hours later indicated that everything had not been cleared out.

"There's still some barium sitting there," he said, "We'd like you to have another Fleet and blast it on out!"

"More fun, huh?" I asked, grinning.

A few minutes later, two nurses arrived.

"She's never given an enema before," said one of them, pointing to the other, "Would you mind if she does it?"

We were starting to redefine embarrassing by the minute; it was kind of funny.

"Sure, why not? What the hell," I laughed.

Let's have a party! Bring all the other hot nurses!

This time, it definitely worked, albeit with a delay. It happened in the middle of the night, fast and furious and I had no control. Definitely not a pretty sight! Three nurses were needed to clean me, two of them helping to turn me on my right side which I had not done for eight or nine years.

"No, no. Wait, wait, wait—I can't turn that way," I protested.

"Well, I'm sorry," said the nurse, "We have to clean you."

"But I really can't turn that way. Isn't there some other way?" I pleaded, tears streaming down my face.

I could not have been any more humiliated. Every last shred of my dignity was gone. Maybe it was no big deal to other people, but it was to me.

At least it was not life-threatening; what happened the next night was.

As I was finally starting to fall asleep comfortably, nurses and doctors rushed frantically into my room with an EKG machine.

"Are you feeling okay?" one of them asked.

I was totally puzzled. "I'm fine. I was just about to fall asleep. Why? Is something wrong?" I asked, now alarmed.

It turned out that I had just had an episode of v-tach, or ventricular trachycardia, a dangerous type of irregular heartbeat, or arrhythmia. The irregular beats were observed on several occasions over the next day or so. It was reported that I had as many as 16 beats in a row at a rate as high as 300 beats per minute. Pretty scary, indeed, but I didn't feel a thing.

There was no clear-cut explanation for the v-tach, but a few logical causes were identified: the weakening of my heart due to my disease, the stress on my body from surgery, and electrolyte imbalance as a result of my "refeeding."

Soon, I was started on an anti-arrhythmic medication. which stopped the "runs" of v-tach. But we now knew just how serious the condition of my heart was. It was an issue that would need to be revisited.

"Relax; get some rest," I was told by a doctor and nurse, as lack of sleep was certainly not good for my heart.

That was easier said than done. Everyone thought I wasn't sleeping because I was "anxious," but the constant interruptions, especially at night, made it impossible to sleep. Every time I started to drift off, a nurse, doctor, respiratory therapist, or phlebotomist showed up. Not that I helped the situation because after he or she performed his or her task, I talked the person half to death.

I genuinely enjoyed meeting new people and learning their stories. If I had to be in this situation, I was going to get something out of it. If I talked to people, they would see me as a normal adult and have an easier time relating to me and I might receive better care. Perhaps they would be gentler handling me or take more time to explain what they were doing.

Talking was the only way for me to effectively pass time. Watching television was useless, as my attention span never lasted more than a few minutes. I tried watching videotapes brought from home, but was simply not interested. My mind knew that I was trying to distract it and refused to play along.

The nurses seemed to enjoy interacting with me. No doubt most of them enjoyed working with children or they would not have been working at that hospital, but I'm sure I offered a healthy change of pace. After all, we were about the same age. I would have been willing to talk all day, as I certainly wasn't going anywhere.

I took a liking to one nurse in particular, a shy but sweet 22-year-old Brooklyn native. I was immediately attracted to her and wanted to talk to her more than anything.

"Brooklyn, huh?" I asked. "But you don't have that ridiculous accent!"

"Well, it must have been all those years in Catholic school. They trained it right out of me," she laughed.

We talked the entire time she took care of me. Actually, I did most of the talking, but I loved the attention she gave me. It almost made me forget about being stuck in a hospital bed. I offered to answer any questions she had about my disease, wanting to help in case she ever encountered another patient with Duchenne. Of course, I would have talked about anything, as long as she spent time with me. She said she would definitely take me up on my offer. Sure enough, she returned a few hours later.

I was more than happy to tell her what she wanted to know, and felt useful for the first time in days.

If I had any anxiety, it was because I was afraid that someone would extend my arms or legs too far when examining me. At home, it often took weeks until I trusted new attendants to move me. Now, there were different nurses and doctors coming in all the time. Every time someone came near me, I cringed with fear. "Be careful. My arms and legs don't stretch," I warned.

Not that it mattered. While I was being moved in bed one morning, my leg got caught and my knee was extended too far. I cried out in pain. It hurt so badly that I was sure I had broken my leg.

Just great. I need something else to worry about. How many times do I have to tell people to be careful with my legs? I can't believe this!

The doctor examined my leg and assured me it was unlikely that it was broken. I could tell he thought I was being overly dramatic, but he ordered x-rays anyway. I was scared to death when the technician was positioning my leg for the camera, afraid that she would hurt my leg even more. Fortunately, the x-rays came back negative; I had really dodged a bullet.

That certainly didn't do much to combat the perception everyone had that I was overly anxious. It was frustrating, and probably due to the fact that I asked so many questions. But I hated being out of the loop and wanted to know about everything that was being done for me, not only because my life depended on it but because I actually found it interesting. I won't deny that I had some anxiety. Who could blame me? Everything was all new to me, and people sometimes failed to explain things.

One evening, I suddenly awoke and tried to talk to Dad, but nothing came out of my mouth. I had been so relieved to be able to talk with the trach. Now, my eyes grew wide with fear.

What happened? I was talking fine before. How am I going to communicate?

When the respiratory therapist came into the room, she explained that the reason I couldn't speak was that the "cuff" on my trach had been inflated with air. Essentially a balloon wrapped around the trach tube, the inflated cuff blocked my windpipe so that air could only enter and exit my lungs through my tracheostomy, ensuring that the maximum amount of air reached my lungs. Apparently, too much air had been escaping through my nose and mouth and the ventilator alarm sounded, at which point the therapist had inflated the cuff, using a small syringe.

"Who said that was okay with me?" I demanded after she deflated the cuff.

Even scarier was the first time I was taken off the ventilator. No one explained what to expect. All I knew was that it felt like I was being suffocated.

I can't breathe! I can't breathe!

"You can breathe on your own," said the respiratory therapist, seeing the panicked look my face.

But it was too late. My heart started to race and the monitor began beeping like crazy. He put me back on the vent, and just like that my heart stopped racing and I was able to calm down.

I was confused. My pulmonologist had told me that I wouldn't need the vent all the time and that was my goal. I didn't want to be completely ventilator-dependent unless it was absolutely necessary. Why did it feel like I was suffocating when I was removed from the vent?

"So you're saying I can breathe?" I asked the respiratory therapist a few hours later.

"Your brain knows how to breathe," he explained, "It's just that the muscles you use for breathing are weak."

I asked him if I could try to come off the vent again, with the caveat that he put me back on if I felt uncomfortable, and he agreed. It went much better this time because I was able to relax.

Hey, look at that. I'm breathing! I can breathe!

I was enthusiastic to learn about everything that was happening to me. I wanted to get used to the way things were going to be, even if they were scary or unpleasant. So when the time came to change my trach for the first time, I was ready. I wondered if it would hurt. Not that I had any choice.

I had to lay flat on my back while someone cradled my neck to make it easier to get the new tube in. The change had to be done quickly because the hole in my trachea was so new and could start to close. On a count of three, someone pulled the trach out and another person inserted the new one. It was a strange sensation, but not painful. It made me cough and I would need more suctioning over the next few hours.

"So how did it feel?" Mom asked anxiously.

"It wasn't that bad, but you can't worry about that. You have to get it in," I stressed.

Eventually, she would be changing the trach and the last thing I wanted was for her to worry about hurting me. It was more important that I could breathe.

The next trach change wasn't necessarily something I was looking forward to, but if that was as bad as it got I could handle anything. I was ready.

But my enthusiasm would be short-lived, as I settled in for the long haul.

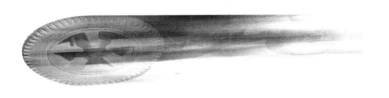

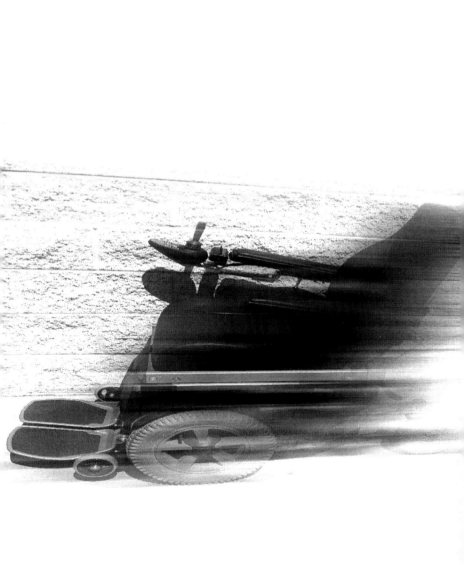

Summer Vacation

15

After nearly two weeks in bed, I was finally allowed to get into my chair. I was being transferred to the hospital's rehabilitative unit, known as the Children's Seashore House. I had spent so much time in bed that my balance was all out of whack and I felt extremely unsteady on my, well, wheels. I told myself it would get better but it was hard to believe.

I had all sorts of wires attached to me. A respiratory therapist carried the ventilator, a nurse carried various monitors. Mom followed behind with my suitcase. My hands had grown so weak that driving my chair was exhausting; I was barely able to steer. We moved slowly, in tandem. "You go first...wait, wait, wait; watch my neck!" I hollered.

Along the way, we passed the nurse who had practiced her enema-giving skills on me. I nodded and said hello, but she didn't seem to recognize me. Then again, the last time she had seen me she was looking at my back-side!

The second we entered the Seashore House, it felt like entering another country. It was so much more subdued than the fast-paced intensive care unit with its bright lights, bells and whistles. It was like taking a breath of fresh air. Nurses chatted quietly at their station. Patients watched TV in a play area. Though infants, there was no crying; they all had trachs and couldn't make a sound. The only thing punctuating the calm was the occasional ventilator alarm that sent nurses scrambling, shouting, "I got it!" along the way. No big deal. Just saving another patient's life.

Mom helped me get settled in. I looked at the baby sleeping in the crib next to me, my roommate. Sitting there in the cramped space that was now my living quarters, I felt like a prisoner. My hospital scrubs could just as easily have been an orange jumpsuit.

So this it for the next six weeks?

The next morning, it all hit home. The thought of spending that much time in the hospital was too much to bear. I didn't want to get bathed, dressed, or get up. I just wanted to be left alone. The nurse dialed Mom and held the phone to my ear.

"I can't do this anymore," I sobbed into the phone, my speech slurred.

But going home wasn't an option. Nursing care had not yet been arranged. My parents didn't know how to take care of me and even if they did, there was no way they could care for me around the clock in the absence of nursing. Besides, I was still getting used to my trach and vent and probably would have been too scared to go home anyway.

I regained my composure after a few minutes. The hardest part was over. I would get through this, just like I had always done, and would be able to get back to my life in no time.

Unfortunately, it wasn't that easy. Even the most positive attitude could not prevent my spirit from being chipped away. I had spent my life trying to be independent even though I needed help with things most people would find humiliating. I could speak for myself, had gone to college and achieved at a high level. Now I was institutionalized, just another sick patient in need of care.

The monotony of daily hospital life was downright depressing. It took half the day just to get up. First, I needed medicines. Then I needed to be bathed, have my hair washed, and get a shave. After that, I had to be dressed and positioned on the Hoyer lift sling. Next, it was time to be transferred to my chair. With the vent tubing attached to my neck, it often took three nurses to accomplish the task, one to operate the lift, one to position my chair, and another to hold the tubing.

"Be careful; my neck," I reminded them, scared to death they would yank my trach out.

Once I was positioned in my chair, the ventilator needed to be attached and its battery connected so I could leave my room. Then it was time for more medicine!

Not that there was anything to do once I was up for the day. Watching TV and videotapes was boring. There was only so much "SportsCenter" a guy could watch and the Phillies sucked that year, so I couldn't watch them either; I didn't need to be any more depressed. I tried having volunteers help me turn pages of books, but couldn't concentrate with another person sitting next to me. It upset me that I could no longer turn pages by myself, which I had still been able to do prior to entering the hospital. Before I knew it, it was time to get ready for bed and I had accomplished absolutely nothing.

What, I'm supposed to celebrate that I got out of bed today?

Being in the hospital made me emotionally fragile. I burst into tears at the smallest things — when my parents went home for the night, when a therapy dog was brought to my room by a volunteer, when I heard somber music in a movie on TV. I was supposed to be a mature, 24-year-old adult male. For years, I had been trying to convince the rest of the world that I was just as much an adult, despite being so dependent on others. A month in the hospital and I had reverted into a baby.

Now I had to prove myself all over again. I wanted the doctors and nurses to know that I was not just a sick person who cried about everything, but someone highly educated who had more in common with them than they realized.

This isn't me. You'd like me if you really knew me.

Of course, there were more important things to accomplish than getting people to like me. The goal was for my parents and me to learn my care, so I could get out of the hospital. Even if I wasn't able to physically take care of myself, I still wanted to learn everything my parents learned. In time, I would know more about my care than they did. We made no arrangements to have anyone else receive training, like my sisters or friends, mostly because I wanted to get out of the hospital as quickly as I could. I could not imagine asking any of my friends, most of whom hadn't so much as helped me with a urinal. Now I was going to ask them to suction mucus from my throat? Why would they even want to do that for me?

I was a bit disappointed that neither of my sisters expressed an interest in being trained in my care at the time. But I think that even if they had offered, I probably would have said no. It would have interfered with their lives and my disease did not need to be their problem anymore than it had already been.

Over the next few weeks, we received instruction from the nursing staff, learning to suction, to clean around my trach and g-tube sites or "stomas," to change the trach, and to assemble the ventilator tubing. We were trained to change a g-tube, to give medications through it, and to set up the feeding pump. We learned about emergency situations, how to check my airway, how to administer oxygen, and how to perform CPR with a trach.

The nurses were excellent instructors, and sometimes also unwittingly provided a measure of comic relief. While preparing for a trach change one day, one nurse was adamant in telling us, "I like to use lots of lubrication."

"Is that so?" asked Dad, "That might be more than we needed to know about you." Everyone else in the room erupted in laughter, clearly lightening the mood.

Still, my care was serious business. Whether we would be able to handle an emergency was a different story. In the heat of the moment, there was no telling if any of us would remember what we had learned. It was a risk we were willing to take. I was not about to spend the rest of my life in the hospital in order to protect myself from something that might never happen.

At the same time, I worried about what would happen if such a scenario unfolded. I wasn't concerned about myself; I wouldn't be here anyway. I just didn't want my parents to blame each other. That was the kind of stuff that tore lives, marriages, and families apart. I didn't want that kind of life for my family after I was gone.

Ideally, I would have a nurse 16 hours a day who would be better prepared for emergencies. The fact that my parents were supposed to be responsible for my care at all was troubling to me. If I was a child, I would have been their responsibility by default, but it was not the same now that I was an adult. What if I wanted to live on my own? What if I didn't have a good relationship with my parents? What if they were unwilling or unable to care for me? My only alternative would have been to live in a nursing home, which was hardly a viable option. Why couldn't the wealthiest nation in the world ensure that people like me had around-the-clock nursing coverage?

I couldn't answer these questions. Although it would have been great to live on my own, I was just grateful to have parents who could take care of me and who could afford the insurance that made even 16 hours of nursing care possible.

Meanwhile, I had to find a way to maintain my sanity during such a long stay in the hospital. After my first few days in the rehab, I settled into a rhythm. I started sleeping better at night, thanks to medication I took before bed, not Benadryl! As I listened to classical music, my eyes grew heavy and I imagined what my new life would be like.

During the day, several of the nurses were able to coax me out of my room and into the public area across from the nurses' station where there was a sofa and TV. At first, getting out there was enough, even if I was just staring into space.

Soon, I began spending time at the nurses' station. I bantered with the nurses and respiratory therapists. I chatted with one about a rebellious teenage daughter, talked with another about her new house, and joked with yet another about her tough demeanor. I was able to occupy myself, but I also hoped that people would see beyond my disease. By talking about normal things, I felt able to get them to do just that.

When I wasn't at the nurses' station, I tried to initiate conversation and to maintain a sense of humor even when I felt tired or moody. It was not always possible. One occupational therapist seemed to have a knack for always showing up when I was in a bad mood. The last thing I wanted was to be perceived as a difficult patient who complained about everything, but I just couldn't help it sometimes.

In time, I seemed to win people over. If *I* didn't, my taste in movies certainly did. From Woody Allen's *Bananas* to *Analyze This* and *American Pie*, my VCR featured much more adult material than the *Barney* videos the nurses were used to seeing in other patients' rooms. As I was watching Mel Brooks's classic western satire, *Blazing Saddles* one evening, a respiratory therapist came in to check on me.

"Make sure you have the nurses page me when you get to the campfire scene," he said. I did as he said, and together we roared with delight as a bunch of cowboys began farting uncontrollably after eating too many baked beans!

I can't deny having a good time with the staff. Even though we were in a hospital, there was always something to laugh about. Everything was fair game, even things like male anatomy and bowel movements (including my own).

Loaded up with laxatives, let's just say things could get explosive when I used the toilet. For that reason, I liked my privacy. The nurse would position me and then leave.

One night, however, the nurse began talking to an aide only a few feet from where I was about to take care of business. I was getting pretty desperate, but wanted to wait until they left the area.

Please go. Please go. I can't wait any longer. Hurry...

Well, I couldn't wait any longer, so I let it rip. The nurse began to giggle hysterically and then I started laughing. Neither one of us could stop. "What's the matter with you?" the aide jokingly asked her, "Haven't you ever heard the sound of someone going to the bathroom?"

Then there was the time my parents brought me fried chicken for dinner. My eating schedule was off course due to my tube feedings so I had them store it in the refrigerator. Hungry later that night, I asked the nurse to reheat my food. As she fed me, a steady parade of nurses descended upon my room attracted by the aroma of my chicken.

"Sorry, guys," I chuckled between bites, "Nothing personal, but I'm not sharing."

My nurse and I joked that they wouldn't have arrived as fast if I had suddenly stopped breathing!

There were poignant moments as well. On a day when I was feeling down, one staff member told me the story of a family member who had been in a similar situation to mine. He pulled out a photograph. "You see, this is why you are doing this," he said quietly to me.

He left my room and I burst into tears. I cried alone for a few minutes, vowing to myself that I too would make the most of my time when I got out of the hospital.

While I enjoyed interacting with nurses, doctors, and

others, I sometimes became jealous when asking about their plans for the weekend.

You actually get to leave this place. It never ends for me.

But I also had my own life. All of my visitors, relatives, friends, professors, my parents' friends, served to remind me of that. Though I was often tired, I tried my best to put on a good face, to be talkative and funny, and to answer any questions they had about my trach. It was a bit odd visiting with my friends in a room filled with children's toys; we joked about it, but I was embarrassed. I had enough trouble proving I was an adult. I could tell that they were a bit apprehensive at first, but they seemed to grow more comfortable the longer we talked.

Maybe my positive attitude was a bit surprising to them, but it wasn't as though I felt sorry for myself. Living in a hospital was not ideal, but it was temporary, a speed bump in my life. While my life was obviously going to be different, there was so much to be grateful for.

All I had to do was look around me to see how fortunate I was. At 24, I was old enough to have fathered every patient on the floor. Some of their stories were absolutely heartbreaking, children in such a precarious state that they had spent their entire lives in the hospital, families torn apart by a child's illness. I could not imagine what it must have been like for the parents of these children, some of whom would never have the same opportunities in life that I had, if they even managed to live as long.

I was lucky that my disease had no effect on my intellectual capacity. My life had really been quite normal until now, filled with many of the typical rites of passage.

All I wanted now was to go home and get back to that life. By the beginning of my second month in the hospital, I was starting to go stir-crazy. Whenever the social worker responsible for arranging my home nursing care entered the unit, I harassed her.

"Free me! Free me!" I called out.

With a nursing shortage, the situation was out of her control. When I finally met the director of the home nursing agency that had agreed to take my case, I learned the agency was still trying to fill my shifts. Although the director anticipated filling my schedule, she asked what my priority was in terms of day or night shifts.

I told her that the nights were most important to me, as I did not want my parents to have to stay up. It was possible for Mom to cancel the piano lessons she taught or Dad to come home from work early on occasion, but staying awake at night was not normal. It was extremely difficult for anyone to function during the day without sleep.

When my parents and I attended a discharge meeting with various hospital staff, as well as representatives from my home nursing agency and my respiratory equipment company, we finally saw a light at the end of the tunnel.

I only wished I was actually leaving, not talking about leaving. What was supposed to be a constructive meeting was more aggravating than anything else, probably because our patience was running out after nearly two months of other people dictating everything to us, no matter how considerate they were.

When the issue of how I would be transported home came up, Dad indicated that he and Mom would take me home in our van.

"Actually, we think it would be safer to transport Joshua by ambulance," someone chimed in.

Dad was livid. After all of the training, my parents couldn't be trusted to take me home in their own vehicle? "Really? Are you going to send an ambulance the next day if he goes to the supermarket?" he asked.

In the end, we agreed to have a nurse from the home nursing agency ride in our van, but I was ticked.

Does it ever end? When do I get my life back?

I would get my life back soon enough, but apparently not without some strings attached.

As the meeting ended, the nurse practitioner pulled us aside.

"I have some bad news. According to his recent echocardiogram, Joshua's heart function has dropped since he has been in the hospital," she said.

With my already dismal heart function, the implication was that I did not have much time to live. It was sobering news indeed, but it did not change anything for me. What other choice was there? Stay in the hospital for the rest of my life?

You know what? I'm going home. I don't care if I drop dead next week, but I'm going home!

That's just what I finally did a few days later. After

two long months, it was about time. All of the necessary training was complete. Home nursing care had been finalized. My ventilator and other equipment had been delivered to my home. It was time to get on with my life. Most of all, I needed a good night of sleep, free of interruption.

Still, a part of me was unsure. In the hospital, I was safe and comfortable with my trach, vent and g-tube. I had never been at home with these things. And as much as I hated being in the hospital, I had met so many kind, dedicated people - doctors, nurses, therapists and social workers — and had enjoyed interacting with them on a daily basis. They had become my extended family and I had been through so much with them.

As we stopped at a traffic light, I could hear the turbine of my ventilator, a reminder that my life was never going to be the same. We took the scenic route, through the University of Pennsylvania campus, across the Schuylkill River, around the Philadelphia Museum of Art, and along Kelly Drive, where joggers and bicyclists dotted the trail along the river. I looked forward to getting outside and enjoying the summer weather, but it began to sink in that I had lost practically the entire summer.

When we pulled into the driveway, everything looked the same way it did when I left. Once inside, however, the house seemed small. My bedroom seemed even smaller, with medical equipment all over the place — a ventilator here, oxygen tank there, suction machine over here, batteries and chargers over there. And stuff all over my bed!

The only question left was where I fit into the picture.

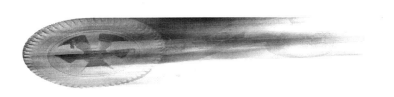

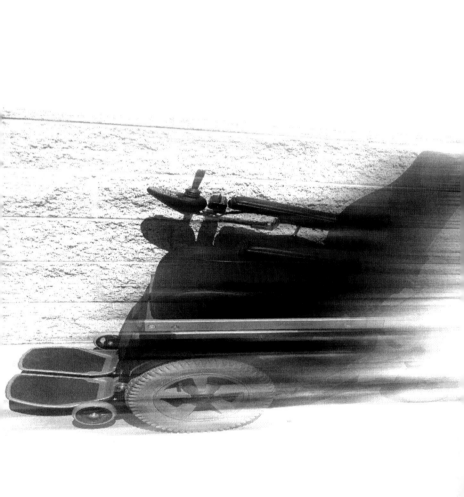

A New Way of Life

16

For the first week after returning from my "vacation," all I wanted to do was sleep. It did not matter how many times my parents or nurses tried to wake me.

"Five more minutes," I kept telling them.

I don't think I realized how sleep-deprived I had really been in the last two months. Now, my body needed to catch up. I slept for 12, 13, even 14 hours at a time. When I finally got up, still feeling tired, the day was practically over.

During my wakening hours I kept busy teaching my nurses how I liked things done, like moving my body without hurting me and using my Hoyer lift. Much time was spent adapting to my home environment. After all, I had grown accustomed to the setup in the hospital.

With the help of my parents, nurses, attendants, and home respiratory company, I had to figure out where to place medical equipment, battery chargers, supplies and medications. A bunch of my friends with Duchenne came over and surveyed my bedroom. Their suggestion was to remove the books lining the shelves. I politely told them they could remove *themselves* from my room.

Those books are who I am. I'm not going to change who I am just because of a bunch of medical stuff. No way!

Personal needs like toileting were complicated by the fact that I was now tethered to a ventilator. Unhooking the ventilator from my wheelchair to take into the bathroom was not necessarily difficult, but it seemed to take nearly as long as it did to take care of my business, although with three different laxatives coursing through my body now it didn't take that long anymore.

"Why don't you try sprinting when you go in there?" asked one of my nurses.

I gave it a shot and it made things so much easier. In time, I got so used to it that I hardly noticed that I was breathing without the vent. Plus, I didn't have to worry about any tubes coming loose. Down the line, I knew that I might grow too weak to be without the vent, but I would cross that bridge then.

It worked out so well, I decided to try it when I got in the shower for the first time. Bad idea.

"Uh, uh, uh...I can't breathe!" I gasped as the moist, steamy air filled the room. It scared the hell out of me.

That was the end of taking showers for me. A nurse showed me that I could wash my hair in my wheelchair, draping towels around me and repeatedly using a wet washcloth to remove the shampoo. An attendant and I came up with an easy system of placing towels under my arms and legs to bathe me in my wheelchair.

I tried to stay positive during this period of transition. It was a challenge — just like taking paratransit, hiring attendants, or going to college. But it soon grew old and I started getting depressed. After sleeping excessively late one day, I had to walk the nurse through the seemingly interminable process of dressing me and getting me in my wheelchair. Once in my chair, I was too tired to do anything but stare out the window at the gloomy, wet weather outside. A deep sadness filled my heart and tears began to stream down my face.

I went through a summer of hell for this? What was the point?

For days, nothing seemed to make me feel better. Finally, Mom insisted that I get out of my bedroom and go somewhere. I unenthusiastically agreed to let her drop me and the nurse at the mall.

"It's a waste," I told her. It had taken so long to get me ready that my nurse's shift was going to end in less than three hours. I wouldn't have time to do anything.

But as I shopped at Macy's for clothes and ate Ben & Jerry's ice cream (Phish Food) at the food court, I felt my spirits lift ever so slightly. The truth of the matter was that for the first time in months, I felt like a living, breathing member of the human race.

To my surprise, people hardly seemed to notice my trach and vent. I had anticipated at least a few stares, but

I didn't detect any—even from cashiers and salespersons. Once they realized that I could talk, they treated me like any other customer.

Adjusting to my home environment was complicated by the challenge of incorporating nursing care into my life. For the first two weeks after my discharge from the hospital, I received around-the-clock care, which basically meant that my family and I lived with nurses. There was never a time when I could just kick back and relax. People came and went at all hours. There was no set schedule, as the nursing agency was never sure who was coming until that day.

None of us knew exactly how to treat the nurses. My attendants had only been around for a couple of hours at a time. Now, we had strangers spending as many as 16 hours at a time in our home. The only way we knew was to treat the nurses as guests. When we ordered take-out for dinner, my parents bought food for the nurse. When I watched a DVD, I asked the nurse which movie he wanted to see. When family came to visit, we introduced my nurses and made an effort to include them in the conversation.

Once we shifted to a 16-hour schedule, with an eight-hour day shift and night shifts, the relationship with the nurses became more defined. When the day was done, I ate dinner with my family. I watched TV shows with Mom and sports with Dad, without feeling like someone was breathing down my neck.

However, just because there was a set schedule didn't

mean I liked the nurses on it. I was afraid to decline nurses whose personalities or skills left something to be desired because there was such a severe nursing shortage. If I was too picky, I wouldn't have any nurses and I did not want to do that to my parents. It was no longer just about me.

As a result, I ended up with a moody, unmotivated nurse who seemed to view home care as a vacation from working in a nursing home. Spending my days with her quickly took its toll. And she had the nerve to say that *I* was the one with an attitude the one time I asked her to do something now, rather than later.

"Suggested to Mom about him seeing a 'phsychologist,' she wrote in the nurses' communication book.

What, did you think I wouldn't see that? And your spelling sucks!

At one point, she pushed for weekend night shifts so she could make more money. As if I needed to see her more. Turned out she wasn't cut out for the night shift. When I called her over the baby monitor I used to communicate with my nurses at night, she must have been too comfortable on the sofa.

"What do you want, Josh!?!" she shouted from the den — while the rest of my family was sleeping.

Why don't you get off your ass and come find out?

After 13 days in a row with the nurse, I put my foot, er... wheel down.

"Look, I know you have her scheduled the rest of the month," I told the director of the nursing agency. "That's fine, but after that, you have to find someone else. I'm losing my mind here!"

With that kind of experience, the thought of having a nurse every day was less than appealing. I felt bad for my parents, realizing they would never truly have their home free of strangers — not as long as I was around.

It wasn't as if I could cancel the nurse on a given day. This was someone's livelihood, regardless of whether I liked her or not. If I constantly cancelled shifts, no nurse would want to work for me and the nursing agency would not want to keep me as a customer.

But over the next month, after I got used to having nurses around whom I liked and who knew my routine, I started to dread *not* having a nurse. It was nice to be less dependent on Mom, especially when there was no decline in the quality of care I received. Plus, I didn't have to worry about asking for too much because I was the nurse's only responsibility, although I actually felt a little guilty asking for things at first. And there was the simple joy of being able to pee whenever I wanted, instead of having to hold it until help arrived!

My nurses were an interesting bunch. They all had different reasons for entering private duty nursing. Some liked the flexibility that allowed them the time to raise their children. Others had become nurses after careers as secretaries, bankers, and even nuns. Some nurses ran businesses, supplementing their income by working a few shifts a week. The older nurses I encountered viewed nursing, not as a career, but as a "calling." It was obvious which nurses were in it for the money (which didn't necessarily mean they were bad nurses) and which nurses were in it because they were compassionate.

Each nurse also brought certain non-medical skills to the table. Computer Nurse had a background in computer programming. Cooking Nurse once worked in food service, while Fix-it Nurse knew everything there was to know about home improvement. There was also TV Nurse, who was good at, well, watching TV!

In some ways, their job appeared easy. They only had one patient, and since my care wasn't too involved, plenty of downtime and some nice perks. One nurse joked, "People ask me what the job's like. I tell them I go to ballgames, movies, and out to eat."

Of course, if something happened, the nurse was on her own, with no real backup other than a phone call to 911. And while night shifts were not necessarily labor intensive, the nurse was really being paid to stay awake, which was not always easy to do when your body's internal clock told you it was time to sleep.

Working in someone's home instead of in the hospital required nurses to balance the patient's need for privacy with the nurse's obligation to be attentive. The best nurses seemed to know when to give me space and when to be at my side.

No two nurses were alike in terms of their strengths and weaknesses, so I tried not to hold each nurse to the same exact standards. Some nurses were able to work extra shifts, to pay their way when we went to sporting events, concerts, and movies, or to spend time with me off the clock.

At the same time, I had certain expectations of all of my nurses, and I wasn't open to debating them. It was my life and I had already made enough concessions. I didn't mind suggestions, but there were certain ways I wanted things done, and I became annoyed every time a nurse described me as "particular." Like they weren't in their own lives?

Everyone is particular. The difference is you can be particular by yourself; you don't need help to do everything.

In any case, I had several nurses, each with a different, conflicting opinion. There was no way I could listen to all of them. Ultimately, it was my choice whose opinion I agreed with most.

Above all else, respecting my privacy was a must. I could never truly be alone and needed help with the most personal of needs, so it was important to me to be able maintain as much privacy as I could. To that end, I got defensive when nurses read things that were left out on my desk or if they pried into my life or asked questions about my family. It was none of their business.

There was no way that a nurse was going to stand outside the bathroom door while I was taking a crap. Instead, I made the nurse stay in my bedroom, with the TV turned on and the volume way up! After five minutes, she could knock on the door to ask if I was finished. I didn't care if I stopped breathing or had a heart attack on the toilet. It was a chance I was going to have to take. There was a limit to which I would allow my disease to dictate how I lived. Maybe the sounds of someone going to the bathroom were no big deal for a medical professional, but they were to me.

When I was dictating to the computer, I wanted to be alone — with the nurse as far away as possible, but close enough to hear my ventilator's alarm if one of the hoses suddenly disconnected. More than one nurse suggested turning on the baby monitor that we used at night when I was sleeping.

"But you'd still be able to hear what I'm saying," I explained

"It's not like I'm going to listen to what you're saying," was the typical response.

"Yeah, sure. But the point is that you *can* listen," I reasoned.

I had enough trouble speaking my thoughts aloud when I was by myself. Now someone else was going to listen to me? There was no way.

And it went without saying that I had to be able trust my nurses. It was easier said than done to trust someone with my life. If I was not confident that my night nurses were awake, I would be anxious the entire night and have a difficult time falling asleep. If the nurse nodded off for a couple minutes, it was possible that she might not hear my vent's alarm or hear me if I woke up and needed help.

When nurses gave me medications through my g-tube while I was asleep, I needed to be able to trust them to give me the correct medications and proper dosages. Most nurses took giving medications seriously because their licenses were on the line. Even so, they were only human, capable of making mistakes. All it took was one mistake for me to not wake up in the morning.

Because I spent so much time with my nurses, it was essential that they truly understood who I was as a person and what was important to me. Despite my disease, I had spent my entire life with a normal outlook, not with the outlook of a "sick" person. After years in the field, some nurses looked at patients as sick people, but I refused to be seen that way. I had a life to live, and my nurses were there to help me live it.

When one nurse suggested that I do with my life whatever made me happy, I was anything but pleased. In other words, I was entitled to do whatever I wanted because I was going to die sooner than other people. My outlook did not allow me to think like that.

"I want to actually do something productive with my life. It's not just about what makes me happy," I explained.

Another nurse said she would be happy if she did not need to work.

"Yeah, people like that are called 'retired,'" I snapped, "I don't want to retire; I haven't done anything yet."

I didn't care if they agreed with me, as long as they respected my right to live my life as I wanted. I wasn't a child and didn't need another parent; I already had two of those. But most nurses were pretty good about that. We spent so much time together that the line between nurse and friend sometimes blurred. I shared my personal thoughts with them and they shared theirs with me. With each nurse, I had certain areas of common ground, whether it was politics, football, or food. And they were with me for many important moments in my life, from doctor's visits to family functions and for fun events like movies, ballgames, and even vacations.

Not that it was always easy.

"Yeah, we get along pretty well," I told a friend. "But it's like any relationship. Sometimes I want to kill them!"

The more time I spent with them, the more I picked up on their annoying habits. Whether it was lateness, clumsiness, moodiness, or talking too much, I tried to accept their faults because my life was better with them than without them.

Still, I grew so aggravated sometimes that I vented my frustration about one nurse to one of my other nurses. Handling matters in such a way was unprofessional, but it was only natural. If I kept my feelings inside all the time, my head would have exploded. Every nurse claimed he could accept criticism, but few really could. If I always said what came to mind, some nurses would have been insulted and might not want to keep working for me.

No matter how close I grew to my nurses, the fact remained that having someone in my — our — home meant they were able to observe and judge me and my family, our personalities and habits, our faults and our disagreements. It did not matter whether they actually said anything or not, but they would be lying if they said they never formed opinions based on what they saw in their patients' homes.

Some nurses expressed surprise at how I talked to my parents. In reality, they often simply misinterpreted my tongue-in-cheek comments. Even if I was rude to my parents, it was hardly my nurses' place to make that judgment.

I don't get to come to your house and do that to you.

But the fact remained that I needed these people in my life. In addition to their daily role, I needed to have a nurse accompany me in order for me (and my family) to enjoy social events, family functions and trips to the fullest. However, such events sometimes felt awkward due to the nurse's presence, almost like "supervised visits." Some nurses seemed to forget that what might have been just another shift to them was something I had been looking forward to for weeks, perhaps even a significant event in my life.

The truth of the matter was that while the time I spent with my nurses was certainly a "relationship," it wasn't the same as the normal sorts of relationships most people had in life. At the end of the day, it was a working relationship. With rare exception, as long as money was at the heart of the relationship, nurses could never truly be my friends. I made the mistake early on of just accepting that mine had to be a different lifestyle and tried to embrace that fact.

Why should I have to settle for a different kind of life? I've never done that.

Even so, it was difficult to feel as close to my friends when I spent so much time with my nurses. My nurses actually knew me better than friends I had known for years.

Getting used to nursing was a part of the emotional readjustment I underwent in the weeks and months following my discharge from the hospital. Since graduating from high school, I had worked hard to become as independent as possible. I may have required physical assistance in my daily activities, but I was my own person, making decisions and advocating for myself like any other adult. When I received assistance from someone, I always felt in control. Even when I was tired or irritable, I found the patience and energy to direct the people helping me, whether it was a paratransit driver or an attendant. Already physically weak, the last thing I wanted was to appear emotionally weak.

Two months in the hospital had changed everything. I was so much more dependent than ever before. Worse yet, I was unable to hide my emotions. People saw me at my worst, when I was tired, moody, or scared. I felt completely naked. The emotional scars of my hospital stay carried over even as I transitioned to my home setting. There was nothing normal about me now. I hardly felt like asserting myself, deferring to my nurses and my parents for everything. I wondered if I would ever get back to being my old self.

In time, I did. I began making the phone calls to doctors. I discussed scheduling issues with the nursing agency so that they were accountable to me, not my parents. What really changed was my way of thinking. I realized that even though I needed more assistance and monitoring, there were ways I could still be in control.

I learned everything I could about my body, allowing me to be in a better position to agree or disagree with what was being done for me. And I took personal responsibility for myself. My nurses were trained to be responsible for their patients at all times, but I wanted to be responsible for myself unless I suddenly became incapacitated.

To that end, it was my choice to be unmonitored in the bathroom. It was my choice whether to call the doctor with a medical concern. If something bad happened, it was on me. Of course, the onus was on me to make mature decisions. If I was feeling palpitations, I did not go out. I was not going to put myself or the nurse in a bad situation. It seemed that I was returning to my old self after all.

Unfortunately, my newly rediscovered sense of control over my life was challenged early on.

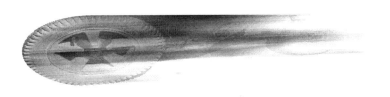

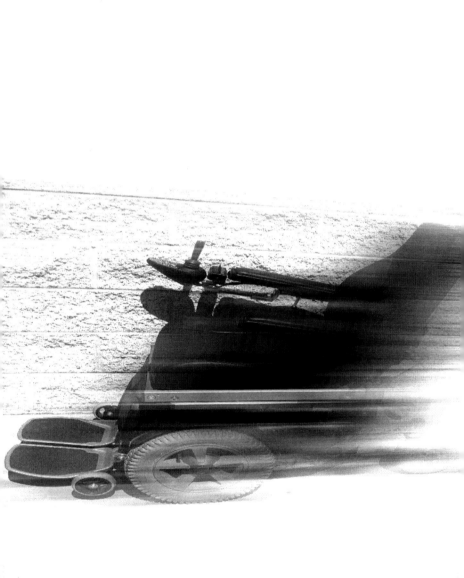

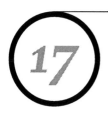

As my nurses monitored the swelling in my legs, ankles and feet, they became increasingly alarmed. I was retaining fluid, a sign of congestive heart failure, in which the heart does not pump properly. I wondered if it was simply due to the fact that I had been given two liters of liquid nutrition each day for two months. I doubted there had been any other option at the time, in light of my dire nutritional status.

Although my cardiologist prescribed a diuretic which seemed to help, my parents and I were not happy with the timeliness of his response. Thus, I switched to a cardiologist used by my friends Brian and Michael. As it turned out, the doctor had graduated high school with Mom. That did not stop him from speaking bluntly in our initial meeting.

"Why are you here? You want to know, 'Is my son going to die?'" he began, looking at Mom.

Whoa! Do you have to say it like that?

The doctor made no guarantees, but he agreed to treat me. He explained that because there was no way to "fix" the heart in someone with Duchenne, the goal was to manage the situation by reducing the heart's workload and helping it pump better. Thus, the doctor prescribed several medications and instructed me to limit my fluid and sodium intake. While this plan of action was common in patients with heart failure, he warned that there was limited evidence that it worked in people with heart failure due to Duchenne.

Still, I did not have much choice. My heart was in such bad shape and I needed to do something or getting the trach would have been for nothing. The only drawback to the medications the doctor prescribed was that they made me feel so tired. Some days, I felt like I was in a fog that never lifted.

I never seriously considered discontinuing the medications, but I wondered if taking them was really worth it if I was always exhausted.

What's the point of taking this stuff to keep me alive if I don't have any energy to do anything?

Of course, I was not doing a whole lot other than going to doctor's appointments, which likely contributed to my fatigue. After all, the most exciting part of the day was figuring out what to order for lunch.

As the two greatest threats I faced were fatal arrhythmias and sudden death, the cardiologist also asked that I consider having a defibrillator implanted in my chest. He told me that the procedure was a simple one and that he could set up a consultation with an electrophysiologist, a type of cardiologist specializing in heart rhythm problems.

I had no intention of actually having any more surgery, as minor a procedure as it supposedly was, but I agreed to a consultation with the electrophysiologist anyway.

When I met him, however, he was less than enthusiastic about me as a good candidate for such a device, and he seemed only too glad when my parents brought up the subject of potential risks. As we left the office, I felt relieved. Nothing that had been said made me change my mind.

Now I needed some time to get used to the trach and vent. I hoped the risks outlined by my cardiologist would not threaten to materialize for at least a few years. If I turned out to be wrong, at least it was my choice. I knew the risks.

Harder to comprehend was the reality that I was in such bad shape. For years, I had believed I was ahead of the curve in terms of the progression of my disease. I had been under the impression that I was doing better than the other guys I knew with the disease. I had more physical ability and never had any serious respiratory illnesses. Now it was as if a rug had been rudely pulled from beneath me. In heart failure, I was in probably the worst shape of any of my friends with Duchenne. Did it really matter that I could wiggle my toes if my heart stopped beating tomorrow?

It took some time to get used to the idea that my condition was so serious. Regardless, I had no choice but to get on with my life and go as far as my weak heart took me. Six months after my tracheotomy, I ended my leave of absence from school and set out to write my master's thesis.

But it was just not the same as it had been before. A small task like reading a textbook was now much more difficult. My nurse had to sit next to me to flip pages. If I wanted to take notes, I had to dictate to him. By the time that was done, I had lost my entire train of thought.

Moreover, my motivation was not the same. I attributed this partly to the medications I was taking for my heart, but a bigger part of it was that my experiences in the past half of a year had made my thesis topic seem so insignificant in comparison. At the same time, my entire self-concept had changed. Before, I was a student who happened to have a disability. Now, my full-time occupation was as a patient and a student on the side.

I grew so frustrated that several weeks later I withdrew from my credit hours that semester, hoping that I just needed more time before returning to school.

In the summer, I decided to give it another try. Though not officially enrolled in school, I began researching articles for the literature review section in my thesis. Once a week, one of my student assistants came over to help with books, taking notes and typing. It seemed easier to dictate to an assistant than to my computer.

In the fall, I enrolled in school again. By the middle of the semester, I was ready to submit an initial proposal. It was not my best work, but I was relieved to have accomplished something.

My advisor's comments indicated there was much work to be done in order to create a viable proposal. Though I set out to make the necessary additions, I had a great deal of difficulty pushing myself the extra mile. I began to envision rewrite after rewrite after rewrite. If I was having this much trouble with the proposal, how was it going to be any easier once it was time to actually write the thesis? With a serious heart condition, I did not have any time to waste.

What if I spend the rest of my life on this and don't finish it?

Sitting at the computer on a dreary fall afternoon, with note cards strategically placed on the desk and photocopies taped to the shelf, I knew it was time to move on. I cried silently, realizing that my academic career was over. Worse, I knew that I would never work in the field I loved.

Then, strangely enough, I began to feel relieved. It was finally over! No longer would I have to beat myself up over the lack of progress on my thesis.

In response to an e-mail I sent announcing my withdrawal from my graduate program, my advisor pointed out that sometimes the smartest people were those who knew when it was time to move on to something else. It was a comforting thought. But even though I believed I had made the right decision, I also felt like a quitter. After all, I had always prided myself on never giving up.

Now that I had left the academic world, it was time to find the "something else" to which my advisor had referred. Although I had spent most of my life avoiding focusing on my disease, my experiences over the previous few years had changed me. I realized that I had developed such a vast knowledge of what it was like to live with a disability in general and with Duchenne in particular, that it would be a waste not to share it.

Therefore, I decided to pursue public speaking opportunities with medical professionals, students, and parents of children with disabilities. Unfortunately, such opportunities proved to be few and far between. I quickly became discouraged, but was not ready to abandon all hope. There had to be something out there for me.

I didn't leave school so that I could do nothing with whatever is left of my life.

I needed to figure something out in a hurry. I always had the answer before, but now I worried that it might be too much of a challenge.

In the meantime, I figured that if I was not doing much else with my time, I might as well contribute to the household in some useful way. With my nurses' assistance, I began cooking dinner for my family, or "burning down the house" as one nurse enjoyed saying. I had always liked cooking when I was younger and taking mandatory home economics courses. I could not physically do anything in the kitchen anymore, so my nurses had to serve as my hands. I could certainly follow a recipe and instruct my "hands" to measure spices and chop vegetables accordingly. And I could surely taste the finished product!

After 25 years of cooking, Mom was happy to turn this task over to me. My nurses did not mind helping. They were there to assist with my needs and that included preparing food if necessary. We just prepared larger portions. Besides, most of them preferred keeping busy.

I also helped out by doing the grocery shopping. Though not quite as savvy a shopper as Mom, sometimes forgetting to use coupons, I managed to hold my own in the supermarket. Unlike Mom, I took my time, enjoying lunch in the food court.

I still had no prospects for a job. Cooking, shopping, and going to the movies was getting real old, real fast. I was getting depressed again. Instead of torturing myself to find a new direction for my life, however, I decided to take a vacation.

When I had my tracheotomy, I assumed that my traveling days were over. In the time since my discharge from the hospital, I had adapted to everyday life on a ventilator. At home, my life was complicated but it felt safe and comfortable. The last thing I wanted to do was tempt fate by venturing far from home.

But inspired by my friends Brian and Michael, who traveled each winter to their family's home in Florida for several weeks, I reconsidered. A major factor was that two of my nurses had accompanied my friends on their trips and were willing to do the same for me.

Several days in the Florida sun might do me some

good. Perhaps some time spent focusing on something other than my failure to find a job would re-energize me so that when I returned, I might have better luck. There was an even greater attraction for me: a chance to see the Phillies in spring training.

But before even beginning to think about baseball, there were more important arrangements to be made — contacting the nursing agency to request the nurses I wanted and to check into any licensing issues in Florida, securing additional equipment from the respiratory supply company, and renting a hospital bed. On past vacations, I had been so uncomfortable sleeping in regular beds.

Two days after celebrating my 26th birthday, we began our trip late at night, hoping to avoid traffic the next morning. Despite meticulously going over the checklist I had prepared — from battery chargers to potato chips — I worried that I had forgotten something really important.

A few minutes later, as Meatloaf's "Bat out of Hell" blared on the stereo speakers, I stopped worrying.

Ah, screw it! I'm tired of worrying.

During the 16-hour ride, I was so wired that I only nodded off for about an hour. It was so wonderful to be out on the road, seeing the country. Interacting with my nurses (my parents traveled separately), I felt as if I were any other 20-something guy on a road trip with friends.

When we arrived in sunny Orlando, I was hot, hungry, and completely exhausted. So it didn't help that the accessible accommodations turned out to be less than accessible. I could not even take a crap in privacy because my Hoyer lift couldn't get far enough inside the bathroom to close the door!

What have I gotten myself into?

"I knew this would never work," I told Mom.

It turned out that a good night of sleep was all I needed to change my tune. The hospital bed proved to be a great idea and I slept like a baby. I woke up early the next morning and was rarin' to go!

Sitting in the stands at brand-new Bright House Networks Field in Clearwater a few days later watching the Phillies, I wanted to pinch myself to make sure it wasn't a dream. After all of the planning, the obsessing, and the traveling, I was finally there. I felt a tremendous sense of satisfaction.

Almost as quickly, I put myself down.

What the hell am I taking a vacation from? I don't do anything.

Still, my vacation re-energized me, giving me a new zest for life. Anything seemed possible. Unfortunately, I fell back into the same old, monotonous routine when I returned home. I wondered if I would ever do anything productive with my life.

By the summer, nothing had changed. So I did the only thing I seemed to do well — I planned another vacation — this time to Boston, a trip I had postponed two years earlier due to my impending tracheotomy. Only this time, I had a bunch of medical equipment and two nurses with me.

The trip was equally successful to the trip to Florida. I was able to get a feel for the city by taking a "Duck Tour," on an amphibious vehicle formerly used for military purposes. And I had the opportunity to watch the eventual World Champion Red Sox at the best ballpark in America, Fenway Park.

Two years earlier, when my pulmonologist had told me to cancel my trip to Boston, telling me that there would be "plenty of time for baseball later," I didn't believe him for a second. Yet, there I was, sitting in the stands with my parents and nurses, watching the Red Sox pound the visiting Oakland A's.

It was not only possible to travel now that I was on a ventilator, but it was easier thanks to the presence of my nurses. Too bad that figuring out what to do with the rest of my life was so much more difficult.

I had no way of anticipating the heartache I would endure before I had a chance to figure it out.

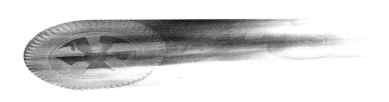

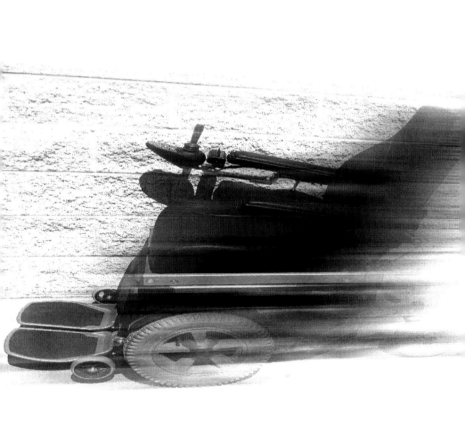

Brian

There's been some sort of emergency with Brian," said the voice on the other end of the line.

It was as if someone had punched me in the stomach. My friend had survived a cardiac scare a few months earlier, but he had sustained serious damage to his heart. Now I suspected the worst.

"Oh...um...uh...uh...I'll call back later," I stuttered, motioning with my head to my nurse to hang up the phone.

I sat at the computer in stunned silence. The day had begun with such promise. The sun was shining bright on this beautiful, unseasonably warm November day, and I was full of energy. It was Election Day, and I was hopeful that a new president of the United States would be elected by the end of the day.

It was an even bigger day for me. Having decided a

few months earlier to try my hand at writing magazine articles focusing on disability issues, I was finally going to put the finishing touches on my first article, a humor piece about some of the ridiculous things total strangers said to people with disabilities. I had even received some interest from a disability magazine. It was about time that I finally did something positive with my life. Brian and his brother Michael had provided a few anecdotes for the article, and I had wanted to share the finished product with them. That was all out the window now. I hoped that my friend would be okay, but had a bad feeling.

Though I pretended to get back to work, I simply closed the file containing my manuscript and began aimlessly surfing the Internet. I said nothing to my nurse; it was none of his business. He hardly knew Brian. After all, I didn't have to share *everything* with my nurses. For Brian's sake — and for mine — couldn't this be kept quiet for just a little while? My friend and his family had been through enough.

Not long after, Dad called me from his office.

"I've got some sad news," he began, "Brian passed away this afternoon."

I was not really sure what to say and I started to feel slightly choked up, but I was able to compose myself.

"I had a feeling," I told him and explained how I had known.

There were several emotions running through my head at this time, but feeling sorry for Brian was not one of them. First of all, I did not think he would have wanted that. Just as importantly though, Brian knew this would happen eventually, as I and others with the disease understood. It was an unfortunate reality, but if you faced it with courage, people would always have respect for you.

Part of me wanted to say, "Sure, this is terrible, but it happened to someone else. I'm fine; it's not going to happen to me."

If only that were true.

I went about my routine that night, but it wasn't easy. I could not stop thinking of Brian and what his death meant for me. Brian had lived the longest of anyone I knew with Duchenne. While I realized that no two people with the disease were affected the same, I felt that as long as Brian was doing well I had plenty of time before I needed to worry.

Although I had been intently following the presidential campaign for weeks, I watched the election returns that night with a detached feeling. All I could think of was what had happened to Brian. The election seemed to be on a distant planet, but I still hoped that the Democratic candidate, John Kerry, would win.

Maybe something good could happen today.

It looked promising at first, but by the time I went to bed that night it was pretty clear that George W. Bush was going to win his re-election bid.

The next day began like a bad dream. Mom woke me with the news that despite some issues in Ohio, Bush had indeed won the election. Then I remembered about Brian and felt even worse. It was going to be a *long* day.

When my nurse arrived that morning, Mom told her about Brian. I didn't really want to discuss the news with my nurses, but I figured that they should at least be aware of why I might have seemed down.

Throughout the day, I kept thinking about what I could do to help Brian's family get through this horrible time. I planned to visit with them the following day, but wanted to do more. What could I do? Late that afternoon, I decided to do what I did best: write. I would write about my late friend, about what he meant to me, and present it to his family.

My nurse left the room so I could dictate to the computer privately. I had a difficult time getting started, but suddenly the words began to flow. It was one of the easiest pieces I had ever written. I continued to work on it until finished, despite the fact that my nurse's shift was almost over and I still needed help to use the toilet. But she knew how important this was and assured me that it would be okay if we ran a few minutes late.

It seemed appropriate that the next day was cool and rainy. Visiting with Brian's family, I knew someone was missing, but as much as I understood the reality my mind could not fully comprehend the situation. And what exactly was the protocol when in the company of those who had just lost a loved one? Was I supposed to talk as if nothing had happened or to acknowledge the situation?

I decided to just be myself. I thought I could be most helpful that way. We engaged in normal conversation, in hushed voices. In between, I could hear the relentless sound of the pouring rain outside. It was obvious that Brian's family was going through quite an ordeal, but the way that they welcomed me into their home made me feel at ease. I couldn't help but wonder how my family would react someday when it was me they were mourning.

After reading what I had written, Brian's parents asked me if I would read it at the funeral. I immediately agreed.

What would have been Brian's 31st birthday turned out to be the day of his funeral instead. It was a chilly, breezy, clear fall day. I wanted to dress warmly, but it was too painful to stretch my arms to fit into a sport jacket, so I had to settle for a sweater. Although covered with a blanket, I was still freezing. My hands were especially cold. And I was so nervous that once inside the church, I had to find a storage room to pee — thank god for urinals!

As I waited for the service to begin, I was in awe at the number of people filing in to pay their respects. I recognized many — including administrators from Temple, CHOP personnel, and nurses from the home care agency. It was obvious that Brian had touched so many lives.

As "Amazing Grace" was played, tears began to well up in my eyes, but I was determined not to cry. The service was a nice tribute to my friend, yet the pastor's words failed to fully acknowledge the tragic nature of Brian's death, and that made me angry. Simply saying that the Lord had recalled his humble servant was not enough.

How could he equate my friend's life with that of someone who had lived a full life?

You play the hand you're dealt, but nobody's life is supposed to be like this!

In his eulogy, Michael said his brother had not been afraid of dying, that Brian had done "everything he wanted to do" in his life. Even with a trach, he had once held a full-time job, teaching computer skills to people with disabilities.

As I thought about what Brian had accomplished, I felt happy for him — and mad at myself.

What the hell have I ever done? I've never had a "real" job. I went to graduate school because I was too scared to get a job!

When it was my turn to speak, I talked about what an important influence Brian had been on me, how I had always turned to him for advice on living with Duchenne, how nothing seemed to bother him. No matter what the disease took away from him, it never seemed like too much.

Seeing Brian with an attendant for the first time had prepared me for the time when I, too, needed to have someone accompany me. Despite needing assistance, Brian was clearly in control of the situation, not his attendant. A few years later, a mature Brian took me and my parents on a tour of the Temple campus when I was a prospective student. He seemed so comfortable talking to people on campus — especially girls! And of course there was the reassuring e-mail Brian had sent prior to my tracheotomy.

I had always believed in going as far as I could in life, despite the progression of my disease. There was no doubt in my mind that I had adopted that philosophy at least in part as the result of Brian's influence, because that was how *he* had lived.

"Brian still went on living life the best that he could and this is an important lesson for everyone to remember," I ended my remarks.

As I sat there for the remainder of the service, I could not help but think that I was not following Brian's example — or my own philosophy, for that matter.

Brian's not here anymore. He can't do anything else. I still have a chance and I'm letting it go right down the drain.

I had two options: use my friend's death as motivation to do something productive with my life while I still had the chance, or wallow in self-pity and despair.

At the moment, I wasn't exactly sure which direction I wanted to go.

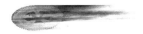

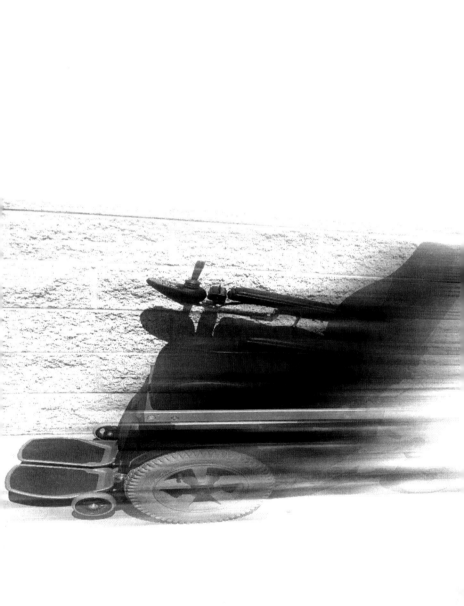

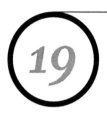

The Decision

19

The last thing I wanted to talk about was my friend's death. So, of course, it was the first thing my cardiologist brought up when he entered the exam room. After all, Brian and his brother were the reason that he was my doctor in the first place.

Ordinarily, he exuded confidence. But on this day, he seemed much more subdued. Brian's death had obviously hit him hard, too.

"You're probably wondering if a defibrillator would have saved your friend's life," he said to me.

Not really, because I'M NOT GETTING ONE!

"It might have," he acknowledged.

I quickly responded that I was still not interested in getting the device — at least not right now. I told him I would "never say never," but that there were a number of issues for me to think about before I would even consider it.

"It's not a big deal. You'd be out of the hospital the next day," he said.

But there was nothing simple about it to me. Other people could walk into the hospital, hop on a stretcher and take it from there. In my situation, even a brief hospital stay could be highly stressful.

Once admitted to the hospital, I could not have my home care nurses stay with me because the insurance would be paying the hospital instead of the nursing agency. In need of help with practically everything, I would be dependent on the nurses in the hospital, who would not be able to spend every second with me. As usual, I would be scared to death about hurting my legs.

I also feared the unknown. With a trach and vent, my life was hardly ideal. But it was manageable and I felt fortunate. I had little desire to push my luck. What if some unanticipated complication arose? If I made it through the procedure, would there be more changes to my lifestyle?

Maybe doctors could minimize such concerns, but this was not something I could just do at the drop of a hat. I needed to psyche myself up for something like this. I needed to fully commit, to accept that it might not be comfortable, that I might be scared.

And if any complications arose, well, then I had made my choice and was aware of the risks. The truth of the matter was that I could not get psyched for something like this right now.

Still, I began to think about it. Maybe it wouldn't be

that bad. When the doctor called on an unrelated matter, I asked him how much longer the defibrillator might help me live.

"Probably another year," he said.

That's it? My life has come down to one more year?

I dared not ask whether he meant another year from now or another year from when my heart might have given out without the device.

"See, I'm just not sure if it's worth it," I said, trying to hide my disappointment.

For two years, I had lived as a patient, not a person. Once highly motivated and goal-oriented, I now had no purpose in life. I spent my days focusing on my health, watching TV, and surfing the Internet. Once a week, I went to the movies. The highlight of my day, it seemed, was eating something good for dinner. This was the life I wanted to prolong?

I had the trach, vent and feeding tube, without which I knew I would have died, but was not necessarily interested in doing anything additional to keep me alive. Even so, because I did not have a do-not-resuscitate order, every effort would be made to save my life in an emergency situation. That was as far as I wanted to go.

If I managed to live more than a year with the defibrillator, I would become a living, breathing waste of space. Not only that, but the longer I lived, the older my parents became. They couldn't take care of me forever. Dad, who had developed his own heart condition, swore he would never retire. But what if something happened? How would we pay the medical insurance bills? And what about Mom, who cared for me at times when I did not have a nurse? I certainly did not want to burden my parents — especially when I wasn't doing anything useful with my life.

It would also have been another thing if some sort of treatment for the disease was imminent and I just needed to hold on, but that did not seem to be the case. Clinical trials that I read about were geared toward young patients with the disease. From a scientific standpoint, that might have been the correct approach, but it wasn't practical for me. I rarely ever heard of much attention being paid to the cardiac aspect of the disease. The way I figured, I was willing to live another 50 years in a wheelchair and on a ventilator. There was nothing that terribly bad about living that way. But I obviously could not survive if my heart gave out.

In the meantime, I was still alive. As there was no way to predict how long that would be the case, I decided to go ahead and try to be productive, even if I failed.

I met with my counselor at OVR, the state agency charged with helping people with disabilities become employed. Maybe I could connect with resources in a way I could not by myself. If it turned out that I needed adaptive technology, such as a new computer in order to work, the agency might be able to fund it.

Throughout the meeting, it was difficult to focus. For two years, my life had been consumed with health concerns. As a result, *I* now saw myself as a patient rather than a potential employee. The more time I spent thinking about my disease, the more time I spent facing my mortality. In the past, when I had been less focused on my health, I never thought about dying. So it was a real struggle to shift gears and think about a job.

According to the counselor, it was important to decide whether I wanted to work "in the community" or from home. Certainly, I would have preferred to have everyday interaction with other human beings, but it was time to be realistic. I would have had to keep regular hours. My nursing shifts would have needed to be rearranged, which would have affected my parents' work schedules. By the time I arrived at work, I would have been exhausted and completely useless. Some days, I simply did not have any energy to begin with.

By working from home I could set my schedule and work at my own pace, exerting the limited energy I had on work instead of on preparing for, and getting to and from work.

How I was going to find such a job was less clear, and the meeting offered no concrete answers. The most significant development was that the counselor agreed to hire a consultant to do a technology evaluation. Even so, because I wasn't currently employed, she could not promise that the agency would be able to fund anything for me, but I was cautiously optimistic.

What do I have to lose?

The consultant wasted little time when he visited with me a few weeks later, almost immediately concluding that my current computer was outdated. A new system was necessary, and we both agreed that a laptop would be a good idea because there were occasions when I needed to be in bed, but was perfectly capable of working. He then outlined some of the adaptive software and accessories he would recommend to OVR. The goal was to create a home office in which I could function as independently as possible. It all sounded wonderful. There was only one problem.

"They're not going to pay for any of this unless I have a job," I explained.

He paused for a moment.

"Have you ever considered doing web content?" he asked.

"Well, I don't know html or anything like that," I said.

"No, no. I mean *content*. Lots of people can design a site, but not that many of these people can write or edit," he continued.

It was a good idea, but I did not have the first clue as to how I would actually find a job in this field. Forget that I didn't have much of a resume. How many such jobs would allow me to work exclusively from home, let alone in the Philadelphia area?

"Hey, you wouldn't happen to know anyone who could use my skills, would you?" I asked him as he got up to leave.

He smiled and promised to keep my name in mind. Even without the prospect of a job, I felt energized for the first time in months. I set out to find an online course in web design — a suggestion from the consultant to broaden my skills. Yet I quickly grew discouraged when I could not find an appropriate class to take.

Damn it! What's the use? By the time I finish training and find a job, I'll be on my deathbed.

How could I get excited about something when I wouldn't be around long enough to enjoy it? It was like test-driving a car I knew I could never own. No matter how great it was, I would have to give it back. To make matters worse, there was no predicting when I would need to "give back" my life.

It was this realization that made me change my mind about getting a defibrillator. Maybe it would give me a sense of security. Surely, there would come a time when it would not be able to save me, and no one could say when that would be. But at least I would no longer feel completely exposed.

Though I hated the fact that I was wasting my time, I still had a glimmer of hope that an opportunity would present itself. If it did, I wanted to be there to take advantage of it. If I had learned anything from my late friend's experience, it was that if I had any intention of getting the device, I needed to do so fairly soon. Otherwise, it might be too late.

And if I got the device and my life remained the same unfulfilling existence, at least I would be able to take comfort in the fact that I had given myself a chance. I could live with that.

I began to mentally prepare myself for whatever the procedure and its aftermath might entail.

Whatever it takes, I can handle this. I know I can.

With a cardiology appointment in a few weeks, I figured I would wait until then to tell the doctor about my change of heart. It turned out that my body had a slightly different plan.

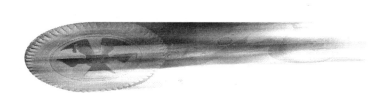

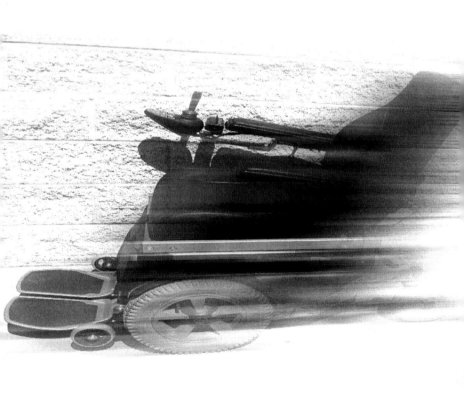

My Super Bowl

20

It was late and I couldn't sleep. My mind was restless, thinking about my to-do list for the next day. More distressingly, my heart felt like it was racing.

I shouldn't be thinking. I should be sleeping. It must be so late. Why can't I sleep?

The feeling in my chest was really starting to scare me. It was as if my heart was beating through my chest. Now the alarm on the pulse oximeter rang for a few seconds. I opened my eyes and glanced at the machine, which indicated that my heart rate was actually very *low*, not high. My nurse came into my bedroom and checked my other vital signs, which were normal. Still, I asked him to stay with me for a while.

For the next 20 minutes, the pulse oximeter's alarm rang intermittently every minute or so, my heart rate dipped into the 40s. Eventually, the time between alarms grew longer, until they stopped altogether.

I continued to experience the feeling that I had initially thought was my heart racing for the next few hours. But every time my nurse checked my vital signs, they were fine, and nothing else seemed to be wrong with me. Although my heartbeat had felt somewhat irregular to me at first, it seemed to have corrected itself. I wondered if I was just making a big deal about nothing.

So I did not seriously consider going to the hospital. With a low heart rate and nothing else wrong, all they would do at a hospital was put me on a heart monitor. I did not want to wake my parents unless it was absolutely necessary. It was one thing for me to have a bad night, but why ruin their night too? I also did not feel like getting up anyway. Still, I was afraid to go back to sleep.

As my nurse sat with me, I closed my eyes periodically without falling asleep. Almost as if I had seen my life flash before my eyes, I talked to him about my successes and failures, about why I had chosen the particular path I had taken in life. Maybe I had worked too hard, enjoyed myself too little, but I had lived the only way I knew how.

I thought about the risks my cardiologist had been warning me about and I wondered if this was the start of that.

What if I'm not this lucky the next time?

I only hoped I had not waited too long to decide about the defibrillator. If I had not made the decision to get it, then I would have been scared, but I would have lived — or died — with the consequences. But I had decided to live, and wanted the opportunity to follow through with my decision.

I spent the next day exhausted and depressed, unable to focus on anything. I just sat and stared aimlessly at the TV. People told me not to jump to conclusions, that what had happened could be anything. But I did not care what anyone said. I knew what it was. It *had* to be what the cardiologist had warned me about. I had never doubted him; I had just hoped it wouldn't be this soon.

Unfortunately, it was happening now. It may have been harsh, but it was reality and it was staring me right in the face. If it all ended today, could I honestly say that I had done everything realistically possible in my life? Had I, of all people, taken my life for granted and wasted precious time?

That night, I told my parents about my decision to get the defibrillator. It turned out to be much easier than I thought.

"The cardiologist still wants me to get a defibrillator," I said too matter-of-factly, "And I think I'm going to get it."

Neither of my parents tried to dissuade me nor did they express any grave concerns about the procedure. I was somewhat surprised, based on how easily they allowed themselves to be talked out of it only a couple of years earlier.

The next morning, I had blood drawn. When the cardiologist called to tell me the blood came back "perfect," I was not surprised, but I was not happy either. To me, it was an indication that the other night had been no aberration, but a sign of things to come.

"Uh...about the defibrillator? I talked to my parents last night and we're ready to do it," I told the doctor.

"Well, it's about time," he said.

We agreed to discuss the necessary arrangements at my next office visit.

"Do you think I'll be okay to wait that long?" I asked.

"You've been okay this long," he told me.

But that evening, as I watched TV with Mom, the strong beating feeling in my chest returned. So did the low heart rate. The alarm on my pulse oximeter began to ring intermittently again.

Not again. I'm so tired. I haven't caught up from the other night. I need a good night of sleep.

Fortunately, the alarms stopped within an hour or so and I was able to fall asleep easily. I stayed home the next day, too tired to venture out. I had a good day and no problems that night.

Maybe everything will be fine.

The following day was the Super Bowl — the Philadelphia Eagles and the New England Patriots. It was a day I had been looking forward to for 12 years. Since I had first become interested in football, I had always dreamed of watching with my dad as the Eagles played for a championship. But now I was dreading the game for fear of how my heart might react to it. It was just a game after all, but I was as passionate a fan as any. I was concerned that I might become too involved in the game and it would jeopardize my health.

I considered not watching the game, but there was no way I could deprive myself. However, I decided that I would watch the game with a detached perspective. If I felt myself getting too excited, I would drive my wheelchair out of the room for a few seconds.

When the game began that evening, I was still not excited. Both teams seemed to feel each other out for the first quarter. I was encouraged that the Eagles came out looking like they belonged. It was amazing how small the field seemed. This was the biggest stage in the world and yet everything had somehow shrunk.

It was exciting to see the Eagles draw first blood, but I knew that it was still early. The score was tied at halftime, but I was concerned that my team had not done more. Having watched sports for so long, I knew that failure to do so often came back to haunt teams. Far more importantly than the score, I was feeling calm and relaxed. Maybe I would be fine after all.

As I took my evening medications, I watched Paul McCartney's halftime concert, featuring Beatles classics like "Hey, Jude" and "Get Back." I felt okay and my team was still in the game. An hour later, however, I began feeling a lot like a few nights before, with the strong beating feeling in my chest. Meanwhile, the New England Patriots had started to pull away from the Eagles. I knew that a

Philadelphia victory was unlikely. I was not exactly surprised, as it was the usual outcome for teams from Philly!

My heart was pounding despite my lack of excitement, so I knew that it could not have been caused by watching the game. As the middle of the fourth quarter approached, the Eagles began to mount a comeback. Now, I was starting to get excited, but remembered my promise not to let it get to me. I now began pacing in my wheelchair, watching a play or two on TV before leaving the room for a few seconds. That was until Donovan McNabb's intercepted pass with nine seconds left, effectively ended the game.

As the final seconds ticked off the clock, so did any hope I had of witnessing Philadelphia's first championship in more than two decades. I turned to the local post-game show, where misty-eyed analysts discussed the game. I wished I could have been as emotional as they were, but the feeling in my chest had intensified and I was scared to death.

Just ignore it. Maybe it will go away. Maybe it's just in my head.

I went about my normal routine, but the beating feeling refused to go away. After Mom put me in bed, I asked her to wrap the pulse oximeter probe around my finger. Almost immediately, the alarm on the machine began to sound. Every couple of minutes, the alarm sounded, often for several seconds at a time.

"What's my heart rate?" I asked anxiously, dreading the answer.

Invariably, the answer was in the 40s or 50s.

I was worried, but I was also just plain exhausted. I tried to close my eyes, but every time I was about to fall asleep, the alarm sounded.

When my nurse arrived that night I was hardly interested in small talk, immediately informing her that I was not feeling well. Upon listening to my heart, she told me that it sounded irregular. She checked my pulse and said it felt weak.

Mom and I decided to call the cardiologist, insisting on speaking directly to him rather than to an on-call doctor, who would not know my medical history. When the doctor called back a few minutes later, I was relieved. Surely, he would tell me what to do.

He did not seem to overreact by any means. Mom relayed his questions to me. Thinking that my heart was being stimulated by the liquid nutrition that was currently running into my stomach, he asked that we stop the feeding. He also wanted to see me in his office the next day.

I wanted to know whether the doctor thought that we should go to a hospital. He said that he did not think it was necessary, unless my symptoms persisted for another hour.

We waited another half hour before concluding that it would be best to go to a hospital. According to the pulse oximeter, my heart rate was 29 at this point. The beating feeling in my chest had never felt as intense.

"If this gets worse, I'm not going to be able to do a whole lot here," said my nurse.

There was no way that I wanted to stay at home and worry all night. I was feeling worse than I had the other night and did not want to make the mistake of waiting too long and needing to call an ambulance. If I was going to the hospital, it was going to be under my own power. If I was taken by ambulance, they would take me to the nearest hospital, where doctors would not be as familiar with my disease.

We wanted to go to CHOP. My cardiologist was not a doctor there, but my other doctors were and I at least had a history there. My friend Brian had encountered a situation like that a few months before he died. Paramedics wanted to take him from his home to a nearby hospital. Although they eventually relented, I was taking no chance tonight.

During the 15-minute ride to the hospital, I kept the pulse oximeter probe attached to my finger. The machine continued to beep as my heart rate dipped into the low 50s.

"You're right. It does sound kind of funky," said the nurse, who listened to my heart with a stethoscope when we arrived.

Shortly thereafter, I was taken to a room. Chest leads and a pulse oximeter probe were attached to me. Next, an IV was inserted in a vein in the back of my hand, not necessarily the easiest task with my tiny veins.

"I'm a difficult stick," I warned the nurse. "If you can get me on the first try, you win a prize."

When the IV went in perfectly, I was amazed.

"Okay, where's my prize?" she demanded with a smile.

As I waited to be seen by a doctor, I glanced at a computer monitor in the room. New England 24, Philadelphia 21, it said. It was a real-time scoreboard. The clock had all zeros on it.

Too bad they can't add a few seconds to the clock. We could still pull it out.

The emergency room was quiet. Not only did I feel awful, but I was incredibly bored. Mom dozed off in a chair. My nurse wrote her notes. Dad decided to go scout out a late-night snack. As I sat there, I could not get Paul McCartney's music out of my head.

"Hey Jude, don't make it bad. Take a sad song and make it better..."

The words seemed fitting, given the situation.

Seeing some familiar faces was comforting and helped to break up the monotonous wait. The x-ray technician recognized me. Another nurse formerly of the Seashore House remembered me from my stay there.

After evaluating my condition, the doctors decided to admit me to the cardiac intensive care unit for further observation, which was a relief to me. A bed there did not become available until about 7:30 A.M., which was a real shame, not so much because I had waited so long, but because the pretty nurse who was going to take care of me had just finished her shift!

Damn it! We lost the Super Bowl and I'm in the hospital. Could just one thing go right?

I ended up with a young male nurse, which was okay

because we could talk about women and sports. Mom helped me into bed — my Hoyer lift actually fit under the bed — and then I told my parents to go home, get some rest, and come back later in the day. As I watched Super Bowl highlights on the news (they were unavoidable), I thought about what a nightmare the previous twelve hours had been.

I spent the next four days in the hospital. It was definitely not the place to get any rest, which I really could have used after not sleeping well in the days prior to my admission. I needed sleep, not just for my health, but also because I needed to have the energy to communicate my needs to the nurses. Most of the nurses had no experience using a Hoyer lift, for example.

Ordinarily, I would have embraced the opportunity to train them, but with so little energy I was less than ecstatic. It was ironic in that patients in the hospital were there because they were sick and needed to rest, but for someone like me, a trip to the hospital entailed *more* work, not less.

I missed my home nursing regimen, which I never would have imagined when I left the hospital the last time. At home, my nurses knew my routine. They knew exactly how I liked things done.

I had also grown accustomed to having my own nurse, instead of one that had more than one patient. It would take some time to readjust to not having a nurse who operated according to my agenda. In the end, I tried to have the nurses do as much of my care as possible and had Mom help me with eating and transferring me to and from my bed and the toilet.

I felt much safer being in the hospital than at home. First of all, I did not have to decide whether to go the hospital because I was already there. More importantly, though, it was the right place to be if something bad happened. I was also much more comfortable with the hospital routine. After spending two months there before, I knew who did what and what I needed to ask for.

Of course, familiarity had its drawbacks. Because I knew and understood my care so well, it sometimes felt as if I knew just as much as the nurses taking care of me. It was obviously more perception than reality, but it was a far cry from my previous hospitalization.

Then, the nurses seemed to be far more medically knowledgeable than I was, and rightfully so. They had taught me everything I knew. Now, I was the one taking charge of my care, explaining how and why I wanted things done. Still, I remembered how much I hated not understanding what was happening to me back then, so perhaps this was not so bad.

During the day, I settled into a routine. I was out of bed and in my wheelchair. Doctors met with me for examinations and to discuss my options. I had visits from some family members. Mom brought dinner from home and I managed to eat. The beating feeling in my chest was still present, but less severe.

At night, however, it intensified, preventing me from getting any restful sleep. The heart monitor also drove me insane, until the audible sounds were turned off in my room upon my suggestion. Every time I relaxed, the alarm sounded, startling me.

Most of the alarms were not of grave concern to the doctors and nurses working on this particular floor because they saw these kinds of issues all the time. I was mostly experiencing pre-ventricular contractions, or PVCS, which were generally considered harmless. But after a "run" of about 20 in a row, I was given a dose of lidocaine, which quickly calmed my heart and allowed me to sleep. I also experienced more dangerous rhythms, including v-tach. I hated being alone when the alarms went off.

One time, a pretty young nurse came into my room. She seemed especially concerned.

"Are you okay?" she asked softly.

"Yeah, I'm fine, thanks," I said, trying to act tough.

No, I'm not. I'm scared out of my mind. Sit with me and tell me everything is going to be okay.

But everything was not going to be okay. My heart was in bad shape and I knew it. I needed a defibrillator, and going home without one was not something I wanted to consider.

The doctors felt that implanting the device was a highly risky proposition.

"Whenever a device like this is implanted, it's standard that we test it," the electrophysiologist explained, "And in order to do that, we essentially stop your heart and see if the device restarts it."

Although other equipment would be in the room if the device failed, he was not confident that they would be able to restart my weak heart.

I proposed implanting the device and not testing it.

"At least I'd have a better chance than without it. And if it doesn't work, then at least we tried," I said.

I also promised to sign anything to protect the doctor and the hospital. I doubted that the doctor's main concern was liability, but I wanted to remove that factor from the equation.

Although I was not thrilled with his assessment, I appreciated his honesty. I wanted a confident doctor, but not an unrealistic one. I just could not believe that I was now in a position where I had to make life-and-death decisions. How had it all gone so wrong so fast? I felt I had something positive to offer this world, but it looked unlikely that I would have that opportunity now. I thought my life was over.

My own cardiologist did not seem to think so, though. He was not nearly as concerned about my low heart function. It was the reality. We were just going to have to work around it and he felt that was entirely possible. He made the necessary arrangements to have me transferred to an adult hospital, located a short ride away, to have the defibrillator implanted.

"They do these things there every day," he told me.

His words were reassuring. It was nice to know that I had a doctor who was going to do whatever he could to ensure that I got what I needed. I had not been interested in having this procedure for so long. Now that I was on board with it, he did not hesitate to make it happen fast.

The next day, I was transferred from CHOP. It was supposed to be done by ambulance, but I insisted on having my parents take me in our van. I figured that I would be more anxious if I had to be moved on to a stretcher. The doctors, though fairly confident that nothing life-threatening would happen, stressed that in an ambulance life-saving measures could be taken if the need arose. Still, I felt strong enough to make the trip on my own.

But as the time drew closer I could not get my heart to relax. PVC after PVC began appearing on the heart monitor. I now began to rethink my position on traveling to the hospital by ambulance.

The nurse could see the fear in my eyes. But she also knew how adamant I had been only a short time earlier.

"Listen to me. You've been like this all week and you've been fine. You can do this. We'll get you up and then we can give you another shot of lidocaine to keep you relaxed and you'll be okay."

It was just what I needed to hear. She did not have to be so reassuring. She could have tried to push me toward taking the ambulance. It was the safer option.

When we were finally allowed to leave, my emotions were all over the place. I was like a lost child, confused and vulnerable. There was a huge lump in the back of my throat. I was so grateful to the nurses and doctors who had taken me in at one of the lowest points in my life and been so sympathetic, so caring. I drove straight down the hall, thanking everyone as I passed by the nurses' station, not daring to look up or I would have burst into tears.

Once in the van, I felt like a ticking time bomb.

"Alright now, drive fast," I told Dad, who had a reputation for just that.

And we were off. It was the longest seven minutes of my life, and I breathed a sigh of relief when I entered the hospital lobby. After I was admitted directly to the critical care unit, we waited for a few hours.

Finally, a couple of nurses came in with a stretcher. One nurse was a real character, with an outgoing personality and a disarming sense of humor. She liked to talk, too.

"You know, people say *I* talk a lot. You might give me a run for my money," I joked.

As they began to wheel me to the elevators, I called out to my parents who were following behind, "Don't worry. This is my Super Bowl, but I won't choke like the Eagles!"

I did not really believe my words. I thought there was a good chance I would not make it.

We met the surgeon, a kind, soft-spoken woman. She showed me the small device that she would be implanting in me. Then she told me that it would be necessary to put me to sleep at the end of the procedure in order to test the device.

"I thought we weren't going to do that," I said.

"We always test them; it's standard procedure," she explained.

"But my heart is so weak. Are you sure you can get me back?"

"Yes, I believe I can. Look, they're going to read you a lot scarier risks in a few minutes. But we don't have to do this if you don't want."

You know what? I don't even care anymore. But I am not going home like this. I don't want to live my life in fear.

I sighed. "No, no. It's okay. I want to do it."

I said good-bye to my parents. I was not upset now, so I thought it would be the best time for them to go.

After they left, blood needed to be drawn and tested to make sure I was healthy enough for surgery. The search was on for suitable veins. It was not easy. They even tried my feet, which was not a lot of fun. I would not have minded so much if they had actually been able to get a sample from there, but they could not. Finally, a viable sample was collected from a vein in the back of one of my hands.

When a doctor mentioned something to the nurse about an ABG (arterial blood gas), my ears perked up. I had heard that the test, which measured oxygen saturation in the blood, could be rather painful because the sample had to be taken from an artery.

"Oh, yeah, that definitely hurts," I said as the doctor inserted the needle into my wrist.

As he continued, the pain increased dramatically. It felt like someone was pushing a long thumbtack into my wrist as hard as possible. I wanted to scream, but I could not.

Okay, it's going to stop in a second.

But it did not. It seemed to go on forever. I asked the nurse standing on my other side to squeeze my shoulder to distract me, but that didn't help. My eyes began to water. I pushed my tongue against my teeth and closed my eyes as hard as I could. I wanted to pass out, but I did not. I could have sworn the doctor touched bone with that needle.

Man, this would be a great interrogation technique. "I'll tell you anything you want to know!"

"Thanks. Next time, it's my turn!" I joked with the doctor when it was finally over.

My body was pathetic. I had become something to be poked and prodded. And I felt so alone.

The nurses began the process of moving me to the table. Once I was situated, we began a seemingly interminable waiting game. The nurses made small talk with each other. I had nothing to say. Their talking about insignificant things irritated me, but they were in a no-win situation. If they acted too seriously, I might have been more nervous.

My mind drifted. I had always had a problem with people who left everything in their lives up to God, but now I saw the appeal of such thinking because I felt completely powerless. I figured that I would live if it was meant to be, but thought more in terms of sheer fate than of a higher power.

Then again, did it really matter? What exactly had I done with my life in the last two and a half years? I had no job and no real prospects for one, and no girlfriend, wife or child counting on me. None of my friends was aware of my current situation. My family obviously cared about me, but maybe it would be better if it all ended for me today and they could move on with their lives.

Finally, we got the green light from the lab. The next step was to start an IV for the anesthetic that would induce a "twilight," in which I would remain awake but would not be fully aware of what was happening to me. Trying to find a suitable vein, the anesthesiologist began looking for areas that might work. When he lifted my gown, I knew I was in for all sorts of fun.

He asked the nurse to keep my belly out of the way and announced that he would try my groin after first numbing it using a thin needle. While we waited for the area to become numb, I could not resist explaining to the pretty nurse that I "never thought that I would not enjoy having someone down in that area."

The anesthesiologist, who had a deep voice, looked up at me and said, "You better not be enjoying that."

"Oh, no, no, no! I wasn't talking about you. I don't go *that* way!" I quickly responded, not wanting to be ambiguous on the matter.

Everyone laughed, and then he began to insert the IV, which didn't hurt that badly because I was focused on the throbbing pain I was still feeling in my wrist.

The anesthesiologist grimaced. He did not think that this vein was going to work.

"I guess that means you'll have to try my neck," I said sarcastically.

"That was going to be my next idea," he replied.

"What? I was just kidding. You can actually do that?" I asked incredulously.

He told me that he could, and after numbing my neck, that was just what he did.

That's the last time I open my mouth.

A green drape was then hung in front of me so I could not see any of the video monitors. I was disappointed.

"I thought was going to get to watch," I said to one of the nurses.

They began prepping my left chest area with an antiseptic solution. I was bored. What was I going to do for the next couple of hours while they were working on me? Worse, my back was starting to hurt.

That was the last thought I had. I fell completely asleep, only to awaken just as I was being transferred from the table to the stretcher.

That figures. Why couldn't I have stayed asleep until afterwards?

As I was wheeled out of the room, my parents followed behind. Tears began to stream down my face.

"Why am I crying?" I asked.

It must be the anesthesia, I realized. Or was it? Maybe they were actually tears of relief. It was finally all over. No more second-guessing myself about whether to have the procedure. I was also somewhat surprised that I actually woke up. For the first time in my life, I had thought there was a distinct possibility that I would die.

The plan was for me to stay overnight for observation and then be discharged the following day. I was not in much pain. Ice packs were placed over the incision, and I was even able to sleep on that side of my body.

But I did not feel safe. My parents had gone home and I had no way to call the nurse. At one point, I grew sick to my stomach and I began to gag. I knew that was dangerous because I was now lying on my back. If I vomited and it went into my trachea, I could have choked to death. I somehow managed to stop myself from coughing. Fortunately, the nurse happened to check in on me a few minutes later. I was given an anti-nausea medication, which stopped my nausea, but made me feel out of it.

That was not good either. The nurses could not have been any nicer, but I still needed to be able to communicate with them so that they could safely move me without hurting me. Furthermore, they were not familiar with my g-tube.

"You just take that tube over there in the plastic bag by the TV, and then you see that line on the end of the tube, you have to line that up with the line on the tube in my stomach," I said with slurred speech.

Then I fell asleep. A few hours later, I suddenly awoke to a loud "snap" and saw a nurse at my bedside.

"What was that?" I asked anxiously.

She gasped.

"The iv in your neck came out!"

That can't be good!

Fortunately, it was so sudden that I hardly felt any pain. The nurse felt terribly.

"I was trying so hard not to wake you," she explained.

She applied pressure to the wound and it stopped bleeding. A doctor checked it and said that everything was fine.

As the sun rose that morning, I looked out the window from my bed and was able to see City Hall. The city looked so calm. I wished that I could have felt as calm, but I was short of breath. My trach had not been suctioned much during the night, and with the dry air in the hospital I was concerned that a mucus plug had developed in the tube. In addition, my ventilator's alarm was sounding every few minutes and no one seemed to know why. I later determined that an obscure ventilator setting must have been accidentally enabled by someone while I was in surgery.

The nurses, as nice as they were, seemed unsure of what to do. The respiratory therapist's accent was so thick that I could not understand him, and what little I did understand seemed to indicate to me that we were on completely different pages. Deep down I knew that they would not let me die if I stopped breathing, but why even let it get to that point?

I concluded that I needed to change my trach and asked that a nurse or respiratory therapist prepare to do so. The problem was that at that hospital, only a pulmonary doctor could perform a trach change. I wondered what happened if a patient's trach suddenly became plugged. Did they still have to wait for a doctor?

As it turned out, the hospital did not even stock my type of trach. I had never even considered such a possibility. I figured that every hospital had such supplies. Although I had a spare trach in my emergency bag, I would have no backup if I used that one. I asked a nurse to call my parents before they left home to ask them to bring the supplies needed for a trach change.

When the doctor arrived, I had to explain my whole story and why I thought I needed a trach change. My parents arrived moments later. After we changed the trach, I began to feel better. From there, the pace picked up. X-rays and blood work came back okay and I learned that I would, in fact, be discharged that afternoon.

Getting me out of bed proved to be an ordeal, as my Hoyer lift's legs would not fit under the bed. So Dad, a nurse, a doctor, and an aide each grabbed a corner of the nylon sling under me, while Mom watched my legs. They sat me up, turned me so my legs hung over the side of the bed, and carried me to my wheelchair. It looked much like when an injured whale is carried on a sling by rescuers. I was surprisingly calm. Normally, I would have had a heart attack, but right now I did not have the energy to panic.

A few hours later, I was home as if nothing had ever happened. Everything had happened so fast that I had no time to mentally process what I had just been through. For that, I needed a lot longer.

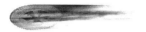

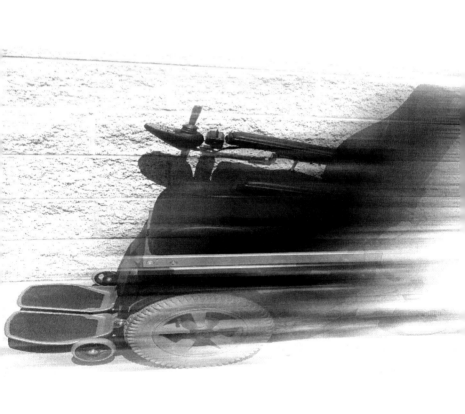

Taking Back My Life

21

I never understood what people meant when they said they needed time to "process"—until now. Everything had happened so quickly, and yet time continued to move.

Wait! Hang on a second! Something serious just happened!

It was difficult to reconcile the fact that I had surgery to attach leads to my heart, the very thing keeping me alive, and returned to my routine life less than 24 hours later. I had felt near death one day, but the next day, there I was.

Instead of rejoicing, all I thought about as I lay in bed night after night was how I had almost died, or at least about how close I thought I had been to losing my life. I would listen to music and be on the verge of tears as I re-played a highlight reel of the events in my life over and over in my head. I mourned for my old life, for a time when I was not faced each day with the numbing reality that my grasp on life was tenuous at best.

I also faced a chilling thought. Because everything had happened so fast, hardly anyone I knew had been aware of my ordeal. To just about all of my friends and even some of my family, everything was status quo. Had I died, it would have come as a complete surprise, as in "I didn't know things were that serious." There were so many people I wanted to see or at least talk to one more time before I died. If I was leaving this world, I didn't want to do it feeling completely alone, as I had felt just before surgery.

I never wanted to feel that way again, so a few days after returning home I sent an e-mail to my friends and family. In it, I outlined the events of the previous week and apologized for not being able to write sooner.

"Please don't worry about me—I'm getting stronger every day..." I wrote in closing.

But I wasn't so sure. Though the minimally invasive procedure had not caused a whole lot of pain, it seemed to take a lot out of me. Not that I had that much energy to begin with, but this seemed worse. Just getting out of the house to go to the doctor taxed me.

Is this how I'm going to feel for the rest of my life? I can't function like this.

As much as I wanted to stop thinking about what had been the scariest and most emotional week of my life, I could not let it go. It was all that I wanted to talk about with my nurses—the drama of going to the emergency room, the serious discussions with the doctors, the nurses who took care of me, transferring between hospitals, the ordeal I went through prior to surgery, and the frightening night after surgery.

One of my nurses gave me a pin with the words "I've Survived Damn Near Everything" on it, and that was pretty much how I felt after this latest ordeal.

As I recovered, I often wondered whether my decision to get the defibrillator would pay off. Would I end up being a waste of space or would I use the extra security to do something meaningful with my life? I promised myself that I would not put additional stress on my body by trying to answer that question now.

I did this for a reason. I'm going to keep an open mind and let things play out. I'll find something. I have to.

In addition to building up my energy level, I had to get used to having the defibrillator. Having committed to getting the device, I was ready to go through whatever was necessary, no matter how uncomfortable or scary. As it turned out, it was not too bad.

I did have to see another doctor, the electrophysiologist who had implanted my defibrillator, every few months. There, information about the device's usage, battery life, and leads could be downloaded from my device by resting a wand-like instrument on my chest. During the visit, two brief tests lasting a second or two were run, including one in which my heart rate was increased slightly. Though not considered dangerous, it momentarily gave me a horrible sinking feeling in the pit of my stomach.

At my first few visits, I learned how the device worked. It recorded every irregularity, but it only took action if my heart was unable to naturally correct the problem. If it took action, it would first try to "pace" me out of the problem, in which case I would likely feel nothing. But if pacing failed to resolve the issue, the device would shock me, in which case I would feel a "swift kick in the chest."

Okay, I'm definitely NOT looking forward to that!

Even though my defibrillator was supposed to protect me, I still worried whether it would. I realized that it would not be able to save me at some point, but I couldn't worry about that. Wasn't my desire for a sense of security the reason why I had even gotten the damned device?

I was also in constant fear of damaging the defibrillator and its leads. There were certain no-nos, like having an MRI or being near a jackhammer, but I could avoid things like that.

Large bumps in the road were less avoidable, but more concerning to me. After riding over a bump on the way to a restaurant one day, I was so nervous that I called the electrophysiologist's office.

The nurse practitioner, in a kind and reassuring tone, told me it was "highly unlikely" that I could have damaged anything. Still, she said that I could come in to find out for sure if I wanted.

"Do you think I should?" I asked.

"Well, you're probably not going to feel better unless you get it checked," she said.

Yep, you're exactly right!

Though everything checked out fine, I did feel better that I had gone. While there, the nurse practitioner told me that lots of new patients called with similar concerns. She explained that even very physically active people had defibrillators, so the devices were difficult to damage. The longer the leads were implanted, the harder they would be to damage because scar tissue would form around them.

All I knew was that I did not want to spend the rest of my life in fear. I started to question how my life was going to be any better. Was I just setting myself up for a major disappointment? How long could I fall back on the fact that I had surgery and needed to recover? These were upsetting questions and I was afraid that I might not like the answers. So I drowned myself in my daily routine, hoping that some sort of an opportunity would fall out of the sky, but resigning myself to the slim likelihood of that happening.

And then, out of nowhere, it did.

One evening, while eating dinner with my family, I received a phone call from the computer consultant who had evaluated me a few months earlier.

"Are you still interested in doing web content?" he asked.

"Yeah...um...yes. Yes, I am," I stammered.

"I have a colleague that's looking for someone to do just that," he explained.

It sounded promising, so I had Dad take down the

necessary contact details. For the rest of the night, I went about my routine, cautiously optimistic. I was afraid that I would be crushed if things didn't work out, and that would not be good for my heart.

But I was not disappointed this time. The next day, I spoke to the president of a small IT accessibility firm. Although the company was located a few hours away in Maryland, everything I needed to do could be done by telephone or e-mail.

On my 27th birthday, I officially received word that I had been hired. It was the greatest birthday present I could ever have received. Though I knew I was capable of the work, a part of me worried that I would not be able to do my absolute best due to the limitations placed on me by my body. I was weaker and less energetic than ever. There was no way I could push myself the way I had when I was in college.

But something was different this time. Maybe it was the fact that everything was new. Maybe it was that someone was counting on me. Or maybe I just felt better. Whatever the reason, I was able to reach back and find that extra ounce of energy that I had lacked for so long. The perfectionist in me was alive and well, as the web designers redeveloping the company website found out. No mistake — a column out of alignment, a missing period — made it past my eye.

At the conclusion of the website project, I received training so that I could make minor updates to the site. In addition to my web responsibilities, my role gradually expanded to include writing press releases and editing contract proposals. Through my work, I learned about an industry that I never knew existed. Companies such as the one for which I worked helped government agencies and companies with government contracts comply with accessibility requirements governing technology used by employees or the public they served.

That included websites. Unless configured properly a site would not be able to be read by a screen reader, a program that reads text aloud for blind people. Images and animations were not exempt, requiring some other form of description.

I also became more familiar with the concerns of people with other types of disabilities, including visual, hearing, and cognitive impairments. For so long, I had grown accustomed to viewing accessibility through the lens of someone with a physical disability. Though I only worked on the communications end of things, it felt good to know that the company itself was making a difference for people with disabilities in the workplace.

On a more personal level, the job offered some unique benefits. Not having physically met my boss until a few months into the job gave me a chance to establish myself without my disability being an issue. Of course, it was not an issue for my boss, who interacted with people with disabilities every day, but I still felt less pressure by working in relative anonymity.

Working from home was ideal. I was so glad not to have to venture from home when it was cold outside.

When it got warmer, it was nice to be able to go out for a walk. Unless I was facing a deadline, if I wanted to catch a movie during the week I could work at night or over the weekend.

If my cardiac scare was the lowest point in my life, the trip I took to Chicago nearly six months later may have been the highest. Since my trip to Boston the previous summer, I had set my sights on the Windy City—and its baseball shrine, Wrigley Field.

In the weeks after surgery, I could not imagine having the energy to endure a 12-hour road trip. Yet I was so wired that after departing from home late at night, I was lucky if I slept for an hour. My heart did tell me to calm down shortly after our arrival. My defibrillator did not take action, as I learned at my next electrophysiologist's visit, but my heart raced and my nurse noticed that my face turned beet red.

I was full of energy all week. I was out all day and still had the energy to go out to eat and then stay out after dinner. It helped that we stayed at a downtown hotel. At nearly $40 a day to park our van, it was a major expense but it meant that most attractions were within walking distance. Not needing to get in and out of the van and having to look for parking three or four times meant we could head out of the hotel doors and be on our way.

I had been on a number of nice vacations over the years, but in light of what I had been through, this may have been the most meaningful. We enjoyed a Cubs game at historic Wrigley Field and watched the eventual world champion White Sox at U.S. Cellular Field. But more than baseball, I enjoyed touring the city itself. We explored the Art Institute of Chicago, visited Navy Pier, and cruised along the Chicago River on an architectural boat tour that highlighted the Second City's spectacular sky-scrapers.

Watching fireworks from Lakeshore Drive on July 4th, I reflected on the past several months of my life.

This makes everything worth it.

I was having the time of my life, and with my job, I had a purpose for the first time in years.

When I returned home, my life continued to improve. With my savings and the assistance of my boss, I purchased an environmental control system (ECU) which allowed me to independently answer and dial the phone, operate my hospital bed, turn the lights on or off, page my nurse, and control my TV, stereo, VCR, and DVD player — all by voice.

Unlike my dictation software for the computer, the ECU required no voice training. Once commands like "TV volume up" or "Bed head up" were programmed, it was ready to go. Even if I spoke softly when I was off the vent, it worked surprisingly well.

"Now I have a woman in bed with me every night!" I joked about the system's female voice.

But not unlike any other relationship, we did not get along too well when "she" didn't listen to me. Sometimes, just asking the machine to dial my voicemail had me fuming.

"Did you say, 'Call Mom'?" it asked.

"No," I told it.

"Did you say, 'Bed head up'?" it asked.

"No! No...you stupid..." I said, exasperated.

Finally, I pled with the machine, "Call voicemail...*please.*"

I had a nurse with me for much of the day, so I had initially questioned the value of such a large investment. But after losing my independence for so long, it was amazing just how wonderful it felt to regain even the ability to hang up the phone by myself or change the radio station if I didn't like a particular song. These were not vital tasks, but the freedom to perform them without having to wait for help was priceless.

When I was shopping around for ECUs, a salesman had told me, "People who have purchased our system say they wouldn't want to live without it."

Yeah, right.

On the occasions when the system was down, I saw what he was talking about. A few months earlier, it wouldn't have mattered. Now, I could not stand being unable to flip channels on the TV or navigate a DVD menu. I felt like something had been taken from me.

Around the same time, I received the computer system that had been recommended by the consultant several months earlier. Because I was working, OVR had been able to justify purchasing the equipment for me. The updated version of the dictation software was a major improvement over the version I had been running on my old computer. Being able to scan documents and read them meant that I did not need someone to hover over me.

The ability to operate the mouse with my head was perhaps the greatest improvement. No longer tethered to the computer, I could drive away if necessary. As a result, I did not need to have my nurses in the same room with me. While they sat comfortably in the next room, I went to work in my "office." I could operate the computer without any assistance; I could answer the phone, and could even turn on the radio for some background music!

Almost overnight, I had gone from searching for a purpose in life to a job in a field that was dedicated to making lives better. I also had a newfound sense of independence.

After nearly abandoning hope only six months earlier of doing anything worthwhile with my life, I finally felt comfortable knowing that I was not wasting precious time. No one could predict how much time I had left, but I was going to make the most of it.

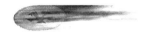

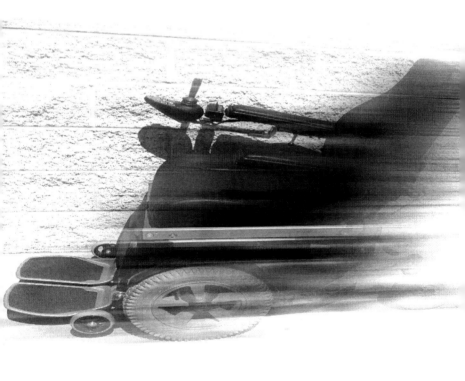

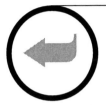

Epilogue

With my job and projects like this book, I now have a reason to get up each morning. Prior to my tracheotomy four years ago, my life had been about achieving in spite of my disease. Then, for two and a half years, my life was all about my disease. My only achievement, it seemed, was in getting through the day. There were some moments of enjoyment, but no real purpose. Today, that sense of purpose has returned, not just occupying my time, but allowing me to contribute in some way to the world around me.

And yet, it doesn't make it any easier to accept the reality of my life. Like the fact that I am not even 30 years old and staring death in the face. A few years ago, dying was the last thing I ever would have thought about. Now I must live with the knowledge that there is not much else medical science can do for me. I have had spinal fusion surgery; I have a trach, a ventilator, a feeding tube, a defibrillator, and I take a boatload of medications.

There are days when I feel so listless that I start to think that my days are numbered. Some mornings, I am somewhat surprised to actually wake up. Despite the defibrillator in my chest, there are times when I feel strong palpitations, and wonder, "Is this it? Is this how it all ends?"

Now when I think of something more than a couple of months away — a doctor's appointment, a party, a visit by a friend from out of town — I no longer take it for granted that I will still be here. I get through the winter each year by looking forward to the summer when I can go on long walks along the river and see baseball games. I cherish every moment I spend visiting with or talking to friends and relatives because I realize it could be the last time. I try to interact with my sisters as much as I can even if they find me annoying like any older brother, because I know that I won't be there for them in the future.

And now, more than ever, I think about the things in life that I will never experience. Despite my generally positive outlook, I cannot help but be filled with a profound sense of disappointment.

I will never have a career. I marvel at people who retire after devoting 30 years to their life's work and think how satisfied they must feel. It is so hard to accept that all of my dedication to schoolwork over the years has been for so little. I've essentially wasted most of my life working for a future I can't have. I look at my friends — doctors, lawyers, journalists and radio personalities among them. Though I am proud of their accomplishments, I cannot help but envy the opportunity they have to follow their dreams.

I have often heard it said that a person should not define himself by the work that he does, but I have always defined myself that way. For most of my life, my identity revolved around being a successful student, I suppose because I feared being defined by my disability. Today, I struggle to define myself, often joking that my occupation is a "professional patient"— and a damn good one, too!

There is also something to be said for the financial independence that comes with a career — to have a place of my own, a car and health benefits. I never thought much about it until I saw my friends — and my sister — reach that point in their lives. As much as I love my parents, at age 29, I certainly don't want to live with them. As long as I do, I feel that I can never truly be my own man. Some may say that having their own bills to pay is overrated, but they have never been in a situation where they did not have the "opportunity" to pay them.

It is highly unlikely that I will ever be in a relationship. I have never had a girlfriend, much less dated. That never bothered me when I was obsessed with my schoolwork, but it is a source of frustration for me today. It truly hurts to know that I am not considered attractive by the opposite sex, especially when I know that I'm more kind and sensitive than most men as a result of my experiences in my life. Honestly though, how many women are interested in a guy in a wheelchair with a tube sticking out of his neck, who probably weighs less than she does, can't take care of himself, and who might not live another year?

People think they're being helpful when they say, "You never know..." but I need to be realistic. I am not interested in unattractive women, so I cannot exactly blame women for looking the same way at me. Every now and then, I learn of guys with Duchenne finding love, but it's hardly common. If that were going to happen for me, it would have been before my trach and vent. I mean, how exactly would I go on a date? With a nurse in tow? So I stare at pretty women. I talk about how "hot" they are and I trade crude sexual jokes with my male nurses. But mostly, I dream of what I likely will never have.

Although I am never completely alone in a physical sense, with nurses, attendants and my parents, I feel emotionally isolated. I believe that's because I have no one to share my life with, no one "to come home to" after a long day. There's no one who looks forward to spending her nights and weekends with me, who has nowhere else she would rather be. There's no one to put her hand on my shoulder and reassure me when times are tough. And there's no one to share my bed with at night.

I can't avoid thinking about that one. Just because I have muscular dystrophy doesn't mean I have no interest in sex — nor does my disease render me incapable of it. After all, having someone wash me "down there" or wipe my ass is about as intimate as my life gets! I regret not knowing what it feels like to have a woman be attracted to me on a sexual level.

I will likely never meet the woman of my dreams and get married. My friends are starting to marry and settle down and I wonder what it must be like. But that's somebody else's life, not mine, I remind myself.

Even if I met a woman tomorrow, how could I expect her to commit to spending her life with me when I could die the next day? Not only that, but I need so much care that she would essentially become another caregiver, for a girlfriend let alone a wife would need to be able to care for me in order to be alone with me. My care is easy enough to learn, but I could never burden someone like that; I have already done that to my mom.

I will never have children. In my present state, I feel like a child myself because I need so much assistance. I cannot feed, dress, bathe or wipe myself and I can't be left unmonitored. So raising a child isn't exactly at the top of my list. But if my life were different, I'm sure I would want to raise a family. Being a father, I feel, means you have matured enough to be responsible for someone else. I am barely responsible for myself. I can only imagine how it must feel to watch your child grow, how it must feel when your child does something that makes you proud.

Then there are the more trivial things in life that I'll

miss. Like watching a Philadelphia sports team win a championship (which hasn't happened in nearly 25 years and seems unlikely any time soon). Or traveling to great cities of the world: London, Paris, Rome, and Jerusalem. Or seeing what my beloved city of Philadelphia looks like 10, 20, even 30 years from now.

The reality is that my life inevitably gets me down from time to time, especially because I have set the bar so high in my quest for a normal life. I try not to dwell on my situation, but some nights as I lay awake in bed I am overwhelmed with sadness and cry silently, mourning for the life I can never have.

But despite whatever disappointment I feel today, I never would have wanted to live any differently. I have no doubt that the best decision my parents ever made was to raise me as a normal child, never allowing me to use my disease as a crutch. As a result, I have always expected to do the same things everyone else did. Though I regret not being able to accomplish more in my life, I doubt I would have gotten nearly as far as I have.

People have often remarked that I have a highly positive attitude. I think this is due to my normal upbringing in which the focus was never on my disease, but on living to the best of my ability. My parents never seemed to make a big deal about my disease and that undoubtedly rubbed off on me. As my disease has progressed there have been times of doubt for me, but I always expected that life would go on. Whether it meant using a wheelchair, having major back surgery, requiring the care of attendants or nurses, or being ventilator-dependent, I adapted because there was really no other option in my mind.

Besides, I just don't see much sense in worrying about something over which I have no control. There's no reason to waste time asking, "Why me?" The better question to ask is "Why not me?" It was a simple probability, no more, no less. I had the misfortune to get my disease, just as other people have the misfortune of getting much worse diseases.

Even if I got a bad deal in the health department and even if my life is destined to be relatively short, I have plenty to be grateful for. My condition is more serious now, but the impact of my disease was not particularly negative for most of my life, due to its gradual nature.

Muscular dystrophy did not prevent me from having a basically normal childhood, from having normal intelligence, from being mainstreamed in school, or from graduating college. If anything, the disease has made me a stronger, better person.

I have had good fortune in many other ways. I was born into a loving family with the resources to raise a child with special needs. My parents were able to afford excellent medical care and equipment, to adapt our home and purchase an accessible van. They were able to send me to excellent public schools and to pay for my college education, which was essential to my development as a person with a disability. I have also been fortunate to live in one of the best regions of the United

States when it comes to healthcare, making it feasible to manage my disease as best as possible.

It is truly the quality of my life, not its duration that makes me most fortunate, especially when I compare my life to that of so many other people in the world living in impoverished or war-torn areas. My disease is a walk in the park in comparison.

I know that my life will never be as normal as I would like. I have spent my entire life trying to be like everyone else, which has proven to be an incredibly powerful motivating factor for me. Meanwhile, I have learned to look at the bright side of things.

My days aren't filled with the stress of a typical workday. I don't have to worry about making ends meet. I have had the opportunity to spend more time with my family than I would have otherwise, including the chance to watch my little sister grow up. I am surrounded by caring, dedicated nurses and attendants who help me get the most out of my life. I have the respect and admiration of my friends, who have not forgotten me. And, if anything, I believe that my experiences have given me a greater appreciation for life and for the world in which I live. My life may not be perfect, but it has definitely been worth the ride.

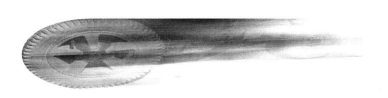

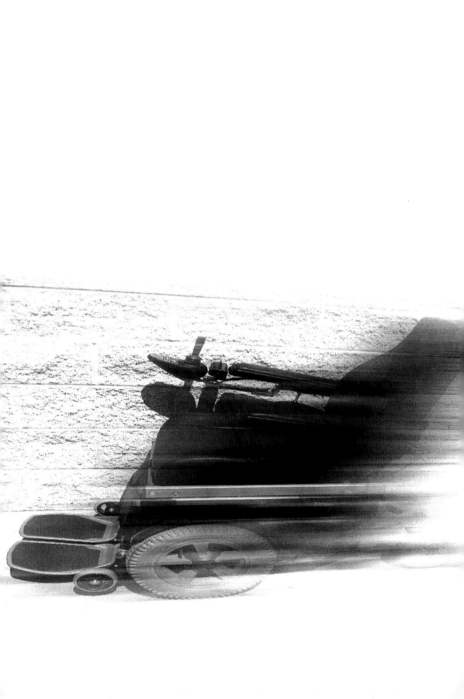

Photo Album

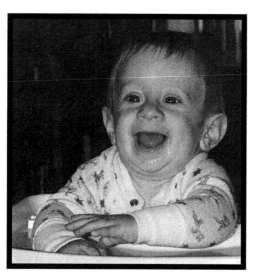

1 Healthy at 7-months, Josh smiles for the camera

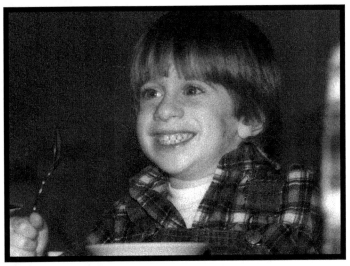

2 3-year-old Josh, happy about Mom's breakfast choice

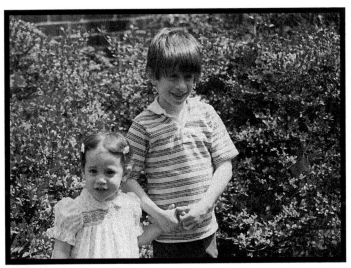

3 5-year-old Josh embraces big brother role with sister, Amy

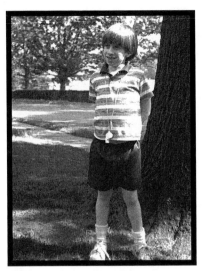

4 6-year-old Josh — keeping up with
his buddies at day camp

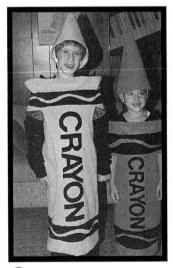

5 7-year-old Josh & sister Amy
ready for Halloween trick-or-treat

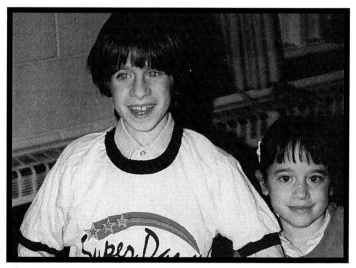

6 8-year-old Josh, MDA poster child at fundraiser with sister, Amy

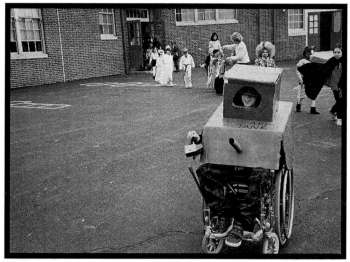

7 9-year-old Josh turns his "wheels" into a tank for school Halloween party

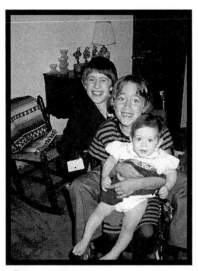

8 10-year-old Josh gives sisters Amy
and Stephanie a ride

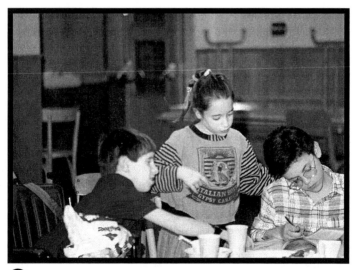

9 12-year-old Josh & sister Amy look on as actor
Fred Savage performs a scene on the set of
The Wonder Years

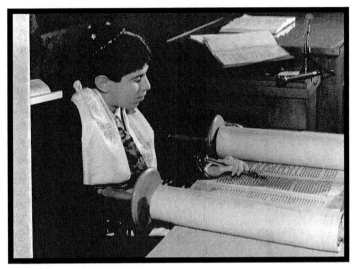

10 13-year-old Josh chants from the Torah
at his Bar Mitzvah

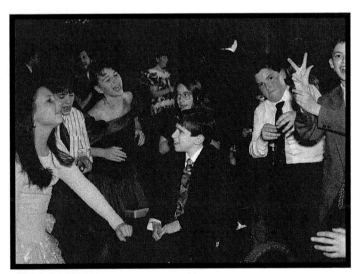

11 Josh celebrates "becoming a man" with friends &
family after Bar Mitzvah

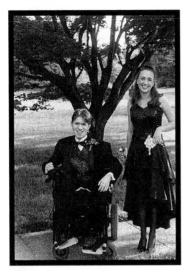

12 18-year-old Josh escorts his stunning date to Cheltenham High School Senior Prom

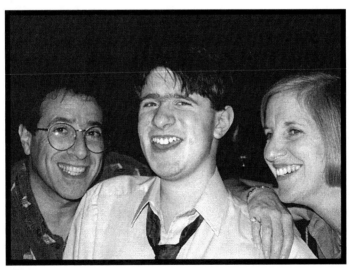

13 18-year-old Josh — happy high school graduate with proud Mom & Dad

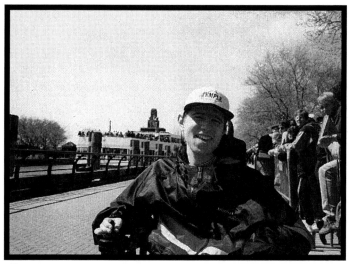

14 20-year-old Josh visits New York City, sporting Temple University cap

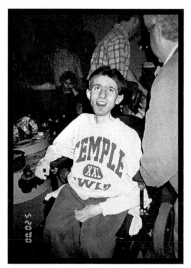

15 22-year-old Josh proudly sports a Temple sweat shirt in his senior year

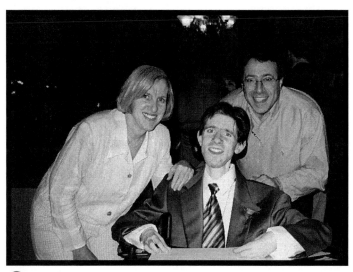

16 22-year-old Josh with Mom & Dad after accepting Temple University Award

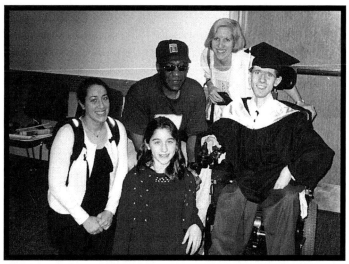

17 Temple University Graduation Day: 22-year-old Josh surrounded by sisters, Amy & Stephanie, actor & Temple grad Bill Cosby, & Mom

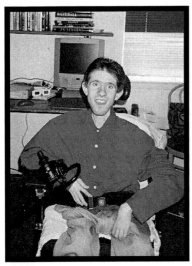

18 23-year-old Josh takes on grad school

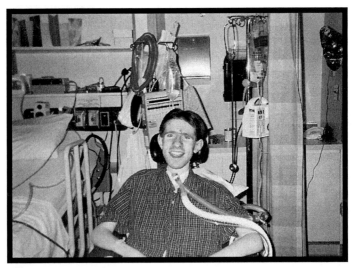

19 24-year-old Josh — all smiles after successful trach surgery at CHOP

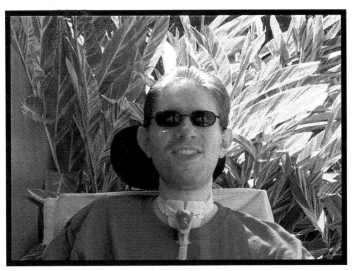

20 26-year-old Josh enjoying Florida's rays during first vacation following surgery

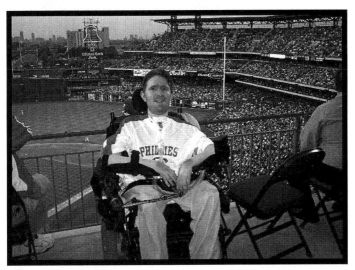

21 29-year-old Josh cheers for his beloved city's Phillies in new Citizens Bank Park stadium

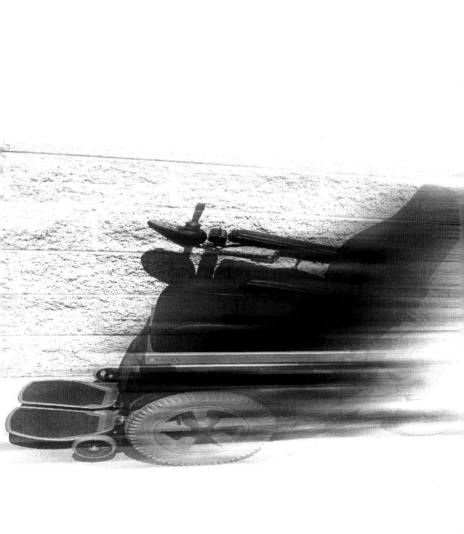

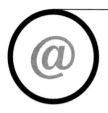

The "ride" through muscular dystrophy is a rough one that no one should travel alone. I have compiled a few resources to increase awareness and assist anyone dealing with this disease to find help, support, and information.

MDA – Muscular Dystrophy Association
(http://www.mdausa.org)
The Muscular Dystrophy Association is a voluntary health agency — a dedicated partnership between scientists and concerned citizens aimed at conquering neuromuscular diseases that affect more than a million Americans. The MDA national headquarters is in Tucson, AZ, with more than 200 offices across the country.

USA- National Headquarters
3300 E. Sunrise Drive
Tucson, AZ 85718
1-800-572-1717

Parent Project Muscular Dystrophy

(http://www.parentprojectmd.org)

Parent Project Muscular Dystrophy is a not-for-profit organization founded in 1994 by parents of children with Duchenne and Becker muscular dystrophy. This organization is dedicated to helping improve the treatment, quality of life, and outlook for the individuals affected by this disease.

Parent Project Muscular Dystrophy
Executive Office
1012 North University Boulevard
Middletown, OH 45042
1-800-714-KIDS (5437)

Charley's Fund

(http://www.charleysfund.org)

The mission of Charley's Fund is to fund a cure or treatment for Duchenne Muscular Dystrophy in time to help Charley and other young boys who are afflicted with DMD. Charley's Fund invests money in translational research — research that focuses on moving science from the lab into human clinical trials.

Charley's Fund, Inc.
P. O. Box 297
South Egremont, MA 01258
(413) 528-5744 or
(877) 436-3363 (877-4-END-DMD)

Muscular Dystrophy Family Foundation

(http://www.mdff.org)

The MDFF is the only agency whose mission is to fund adaptive equipment. From wheelchairs to van lifts to communication devices and beyond, this agency helps you get the equipment needed to live with No Boundaries.®

Muscular Dystrophy Family Foundation
3951 N. Meridian Street, Suite 100
Indianapolis, IN 46208
Toll Free: (800) 544-1213

Muscular Dystrophy Campaign

(http://www.muscular-dystrophy.org)

The Muscular Dystrophy Campaign is the only UK charity focusing on all muscular dystrophies and allied disorders. This charitable organization has pioneered the search for treatments and cures for over 45 years, and also provides practical, medical and emotional support for people affected by the conditions.

Muscular Dystrophy Campaign
0800 652 6352 (freephone)
61 Southwark Street
London
SE1 0HL

HealthTouch

(http://www.healthtouch.com)

HealthTouch Online for Better Help provides genetic information about Duchenne muscular dystrophy; diagnosis, early & late phase symptoms, medical treatment, vitamins and natural medicines. This site also provides a link to a General Health Resource Directory.

> National Society of Genetic Counselors
> 401 N. Michigan Avenue
> Chicago, IL 60611
> 312-321-6834
> www.nsgc.org

Cure Duchenne Muscular Dystrophy

(http://www.cureduchenne.org/home.html)

Our efforts are targeted. We have the leading scientists in the world helping us to determine the most viable research projects...and moreover... to accelerate the clinical trial process and bring potential life-saving drugs to help this generation of Duchenne boys. Our VISION is our name...to cure Duchenne muscular dystrophy. We are dedicated to be out of business in ten years ... with your help. Our MISSION is to save THIS generation of Duchenne boys.

> CureDuchenne
> 3334 E. Coast Hwy. #157
> Corona Del Mar, CA 92625
> 949-721-4063
> Debra.CureDuchenne@adelphia.net

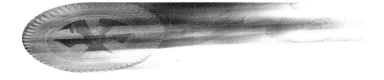

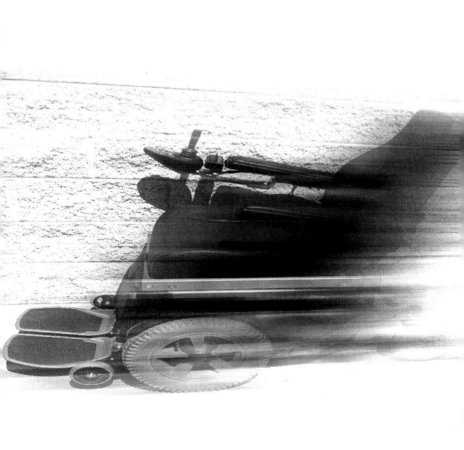

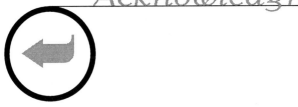

Acknowledgments

I'dlike to express my gratitude to Little Treasure Books for the opportunity to tell my story and to Amy Saggiomo for bringing it to their attention. Thank you NBC (Philadelphia) television reporter, Cherie Bank who followed my journey since I was a child and who became a very special friend. I also thank Pat Furlong and Parent Project Muscular Dystrophy for their support in making this book possible.

Thanks to Justin Vitiello, Frank Freudberg, and Rabbi Lance Sussman for their helpful feedback throughout the writing process. For invaluable medical information, my appreciation goes to Stanley Goren, MD, Kenneth Fischbeck, MD, Richard Finkel, MD, Eniko Kovats, MD, Hank Mayer, MD, Susan Miller, MD, Cherie Debrest, Livija Medne, and Laurie Miske.

For expressing their observations about me, I thank my former teachers and advisers, Dorothy Cebula, Renee

Kirby, Linda Chorney, Dieter Forster, Ruth Ost, and Ed Massa, as well as former colleagues Myrtle Jackson and Barbara Von Franzke.

For sharing their memories, editing skills and encouragement, my heartfelt gratitude goes to my family and friends: Linda and Michael Winheld, Amy Winheld, Stephanie Winheld, Bill Goldstein, Sally Rosen, Steve Goldstein, Sue Gordon, Susi Peltzman, Beverly Ristine, Alexis Carroll, Tracey Epley, Rob Orkin, Marc Miller, Lauren Rosenthal, Kristen Graham, Dan Hargreaves, Krysta Pellegrino; and Sarah Redelheim, who came up with the perfect title for this book; and Emma Findlater for singlehandedly keeping me sane during the final stages of this project.

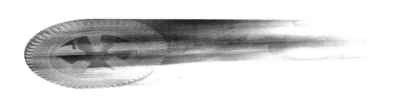

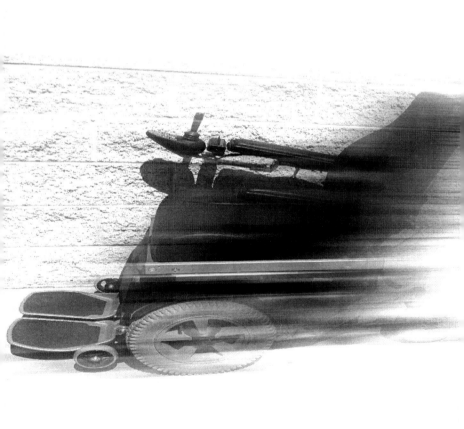

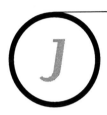

The Author

Josh Winheld was born on March 4, 1978, a healthy boy by all appearances. Less than five years later, he was diagnosed with Duchenne muscular dystrophy, a sex-linked disorder that primarily affects boys. This terminal disease causes the skeletal and heart muscles to progressively weaken, leaving most boys wheelchair bound by their teens. There is no treatment or cure for this disease, and it is predicted that patients will die before reaching 30. Not one to be easily overcome by obstacles, Josh Winheld chose to live life as "normally" as possible, was mainstreamed through schools and went on to graduate summa cum laude from Temple University. Now that he has completed his autobiography, Josh is working towards earning his master's degree.